BASIC NURSING

By the same Authors

A GUIDE TO MEDICAL AND SURGICAL NURSING

Second Edition. 244 pp. 8½ × 5½. 44 illustrations
£1 15s. net (£1.75) hard covers
£1 10s. net (£1.50) limp covers

A HISTORY OF THE GENERAL NURSING
COUNCIL FOR ENGLAND AND WALES

1919–1969. 312 pp. 8½ × 5½.
19 illustrations. £3 10s. net (£3.50)

BASIC NURSING

BY

EVE R. D. BENDALL

Ac. Dip. Ed., R.N.T.

Examiner to the General Nursing Council for England and Wales

and

ELIZABETH RAYBOULD

S.R.N., Pt. I Cert. C.M.B., R.N.T.

Examiner to the General Nursing Council for England and Wales
Principal Tutor, The Charing Cross Hospitals School of Nursing, London

THIRD EDITION

With 48 Illustrations

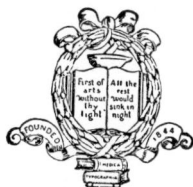

LONDON
H. K. LEWIS & Co. Ltd.
1970

First Edition, 1963
Reprinted, 1964
Second Edition, 1965
Reprinted, 1966
Third Edition, 1970

©

H. K. LEWIS & Co. Ltd.
1963, 1965, 1970

SBN 0 7186 0329 X

PRINTED IN GREAT BRITAIN
BY HAZELL WATSON AND VINEY, LTD., AYLESBURY, BUCKS

PREFACE TO THIRD EDITION

Once again we have to thank those of our colleagues who have helped with this edition, including Miss M. Lee, Miss P. Magrath, Miss O. Morgan, Miss S. Phillips, and the staff of the Department of Medical Photography at Charing Cross Hospital for new photographs, and the Board of Governors for permission to use them. As always we are indebted to our publishers for their help and advice.

E. R. D. B.
E. R.

PREFACE TO THE FIRST EDITION

The term "Basic Nursing" means different things to different people. In this book we have attempted to provide a foundation on which any nurse in training may build. To us it seems that all sick people have certain common needs, whatever their complaint and wherever they are nursed, and it is the nurses' function to satisfy these needs. How this is done varies in detail from ward to ward and hospital to hospital, and because of this we have tried to stress the general principles of the patient's care, rather than the details of the equipment used. We have also omitted lists and photographs of trays and trolleys, since these are usually described in detail, both by the staff of the individual Schools of Nursing and in the hospital procedure books.

We are indebted to many of our friends and colleagues for their help, advice and criticism, especially Miss V. Hunt and Miss B. I. R. Dodwell for reading the text, Miss E. Mann for help with the illustrations, Mrs. B. Hinde for typing the manuscript, the Department of Medical Photography Charing Cross Hospital for many of the photographs and the Board of Governors for permission to use them, the Board of Governors of the United Sheffield Hospitals for permission to publish photograph 48, and Messrs. H. K. Lewis & Co. Ltd. for their help and advice.

We are particularly grateful to Miss Doreen Hayward for her unfailing interest, patience and encouragement, and to Miss J. B. Price and Miss H. Evans, not only for their interest in this book but for all they tried to teach us during a very happy period on the staff of the United Sheffield Hospitals' School of Nursing.

EVE R. D. BENDALL
E. RAYBOULD

CONTENTS

BASIC NURSING

Chapter I

INTRODUCTION

THE HOSPITAL SERVICE

From the early Middle Ages the care of the sick was mainly in the hands of the religious orders, both in this country and on the Continent. To begin with there was little differentiation—the poor, the old, the orphans and the sick being cared for together as part of the duties of the religious; the basis of care lay in Christian devotion and not in scientific treatment.

Later, in about the 12th century, special buildings—the early hospitals—were set apart for the sick, and the *nursing orders* came into being. These were the military orders, whose origins can be found in the Crusades and of whom a famous example is the Knights Hospitallers of St. John of Jerusalem; the regular orders, whose Sisters came from various religious communities which also controlled the hospitals—an example being the Augustinian Sisters of the Hôtel-Dieu in Paris; and the secular orders, which consisted of lay workers with a deep religious conviction, but not bound by the vows of a religious community, such as the Order of the Holy Ghost whose members worked in hospitals in France, Germany and Italy.

Apart from this, it is obvious that the care of the sick at home was normally the responsibility of the women of the household, and some medical knowledge was regarded as part of the "know how" of every housewife.

In England a sudden change occurred in the 16th century, when Henry VIII dissolved the monasteries, so virtually closing all the existing hospitals. With the scattering of the religious communities the civil authorities were faced for the first time with the responsibility of the sick and poor, and the City of London took control of four of the existing monastic buildings —St. Bartholomew's and St. Thomas's for the physically sick; Bethlehem for the mentally ill; Christ's for the orphans and abandoned children; and later, Bridewell—a palace—was pre-

1

sented by Edward VI, and was used to house criminals and vagabonds. From then on, with a few exceptions, the control of hospitals in this country has been in the hands of lay authority.

On the Continent lay management came into being in a slower and less dramatic fashion; in many cases, the nurses were still religious Sisters, but lay staff were gradually introduced. However, the tradition of religious control can be seen far more clearly in parts of the Continent than in this country.

Few new hospitals were built in England until the 18th century, when as a result of a new feeling of responsibility on the part of the more educated sections of the community, a period of great activity began. A few names and dates will indicate the great upsurge of building which took place all over the country:

Westminster Hospital	1719
Guy's Hospital	1725
St. George's Hospital	1733
Liverpool Royal Infirmary	1749
Manchester Royal Infirmary	1753
Sheffield Royal Infirmary	1797

These were the *voluntary* hospitals, built and maintained by public subscription and endowment. Their main aim was to care for the sick poor, who could not afford to pay, and in many cases the reasons for admission were still social rather than medical. However, the need was far greater than the existing hospitals could meet; in 1850 it is probable that less than 8,000 patients were accommodated in voluntary hospitals, though this rose to nearly 20,000 by 1880.

The great bulk of the sick poor were still housed in workhouses which had been set up under the Elizabethan Poor Law, to care for all the parish paupers whether aged, mentally ill, physically sick or merely destitute. Gradually during the 19th century sick wards or infirmaries separated the sick from other workhouse inmates, and in some cases richer local authorities built new hospitals. These hospitals and the Poor Law Infirmaries catered for those living in their area and in most cases patients who were able paid for their treatment according to their income, with charges varying from one authority to another.

During the 19th century few well-to-do people ever became patients in hospital; if they were ill, they employed nurses to look after them at home and there was never any suggestion that treatment in hospital had any advantage over care at home.

In the second half of the 19th century the revolution in nursing occurred and at the same time there was a rapid growth in municipal and cottage hospitals. Developments in surgery and anaesthetics followed the turn of the century, but hospitals were still regarded with suspicion by many, and it was not until the First World War, when soldiers and officers alike benefited from hospital treatment, that the attitude began to alter. After the war it was found that a change had occurred and even the well-to-do were demanding hospital treatment when they were ill.

Between the wars medical science advanced at an ever-increasing rate, and the cost of hospital services also grew. The standards of care varied enormously throughout the country, ranging from the large London teaching hospitals at one end of the scale, to the newly up-graded Poor Law Infirmaries (now hospitals under the local authorities) at the other. With the outbreak of the Second World War, the Ministry of Health instituted the Emergency Medical Services, which built new hospitals and enlarged existing ones. Since many hospitals were coping with military as well as increased civilian sick, it was necessary for them to receive financial aid from the Treasury. With the end of the war, it was obvious that individual hospitals could no longer provide adequate modern treatment without continuing to receive financial help.

On the 5th July 1948 the National Health Service came into being. This meant that for the first time in our history the nation's health and most of the hospitals became the responsibility of the State.

The Government department most closely concerned is the Department of Health and Social Security[1] with the Secretary of State at its head. He is advised by a Council, the Central Health Services Council. The members are doctors, nurses, pharmicists, dental practitioners and others connected with the medical profession and hospital administration. They in turn are advised by various specialist committees, the Standing Advisory Committees.

[1] Previously called the Ministry of Health.

Other Government departments are concerned in some way with health and welfare, an example being the Home Office, under whose administration Children's Officers are responsible for the welfare of deprived children.

The National Health Service Act is a long and complicated document, containing six main parts and numerous schedules of administrative detail. The diagram indicates its main divisions

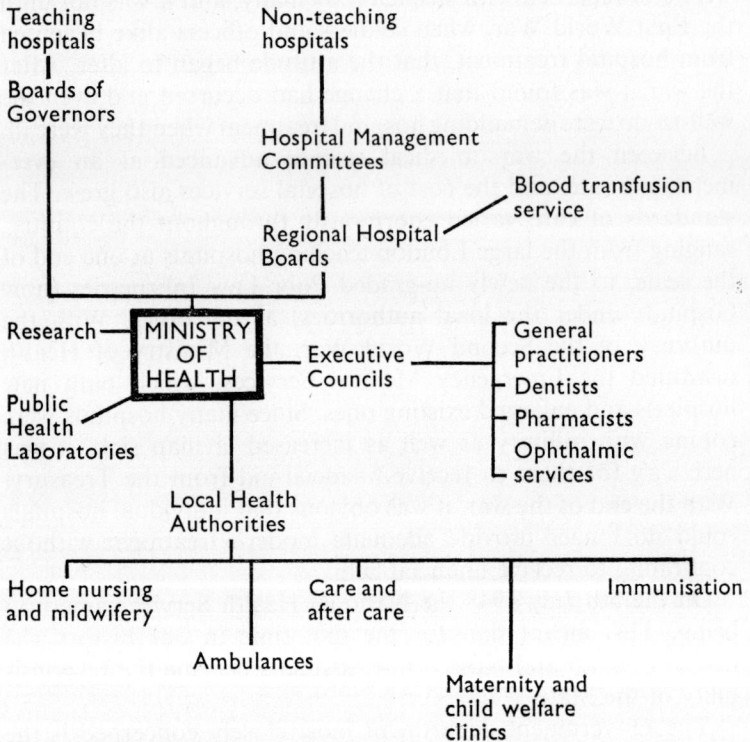

FIG. I. THE NATIONAL HEALTH SERVICE ACT 1946

England and Wales are divided into 15 Regions, the hospitals in each being administered by a Regional Hospital Board, responsible to the Secretary of State. As each Region contains a large number of hospitals of different sizes and types, the day-to-day running is supervised by Hospital Management Com-

4

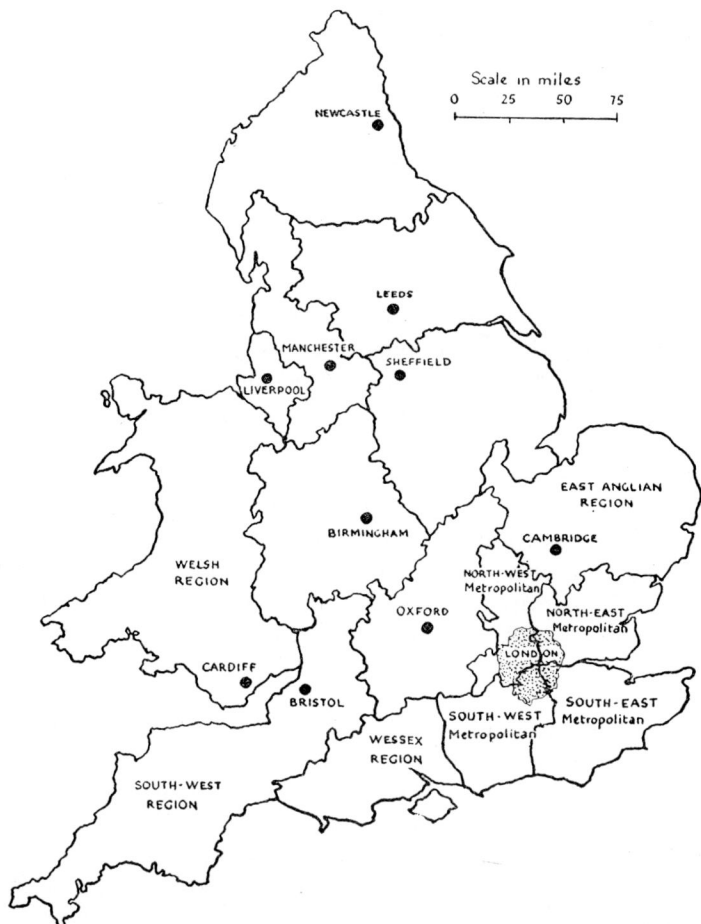

Fig. 2.—Regions in England and Wales. The unnamed regions are called after the University towns they contain (*from "Preventive Medicine and Public Health" by F. Grundy*).

mittees responsible for one or more hospitals. These Committees are answerable to the Regional Hospital Board and, through it, to the Secretary of State. The members of these two bodies are appointed by the Secretary of State, either because of their specialist knowledge, or their local standing and experience. Doctors and nurses may be asked to serve. All hospitals under the Regional Hospital Board are designated *non-teaching* hospitals.

Within each Region is a University town or city which has a medical school. Linked to this are one or more hospitals, where the students obtain their clinical experience; because of this they are designated *teaching hospitals*. They are administered by Boards of Governors who are directly responsible to the Secretary of State. In each of the four Metropolitan Regions there are several medical schools.

In Scotland and Northern Ireland the administration is somewhat different.

During 1968 and 1969 several reports were published containing proposals which, if implemented, will radically change the structure of the Health Service, the personal social services and medical education.[1]

The cost of the National Health Service for the country as a whole is now approximately £1,450,000,000 per annum, having risen each year since its inception: the hospital service accounts for a large proportion of this amount. In addition to maintaining the present level of service, new hospitals are urgently needed as the vast majority are over 100 years old and quite unsuitable for the practice of modern medicine and surgery. In 1962, a building programme was announced, and although the original plan has not been adhered to, some new hospitals are being built and others modernised. It is difficult to give an average figure for the cost of a new hospital, but one with 600–800 beds could cost at least £12,000,000. It is obvious from this that the maintenance of health is an expensive item in the nation's budget. The money comes from direct and indirect taxation and local rates. Although we speak of our *free* health service, it is in fact only free in so far as no bills are presented to the patient after a period of treatment at home or in hospital.

A hospital is made up of many wards and departments. The departments include Out-Patients, Casualty, Operating Theatre, X-ray, Physiotherapy and many others. Hospital wards differ in their layout. The majority of British hospitals are still based on the *open-ward* plan, many being inconvenient, particularly as regards sanitary annexes and accommodation for patients who are able to get up. When these hospitals were built the

---

[1] The Seebohm Report (HMSO, 1968); The Royal Commission on Medical Education (HMSO, 1968).

6

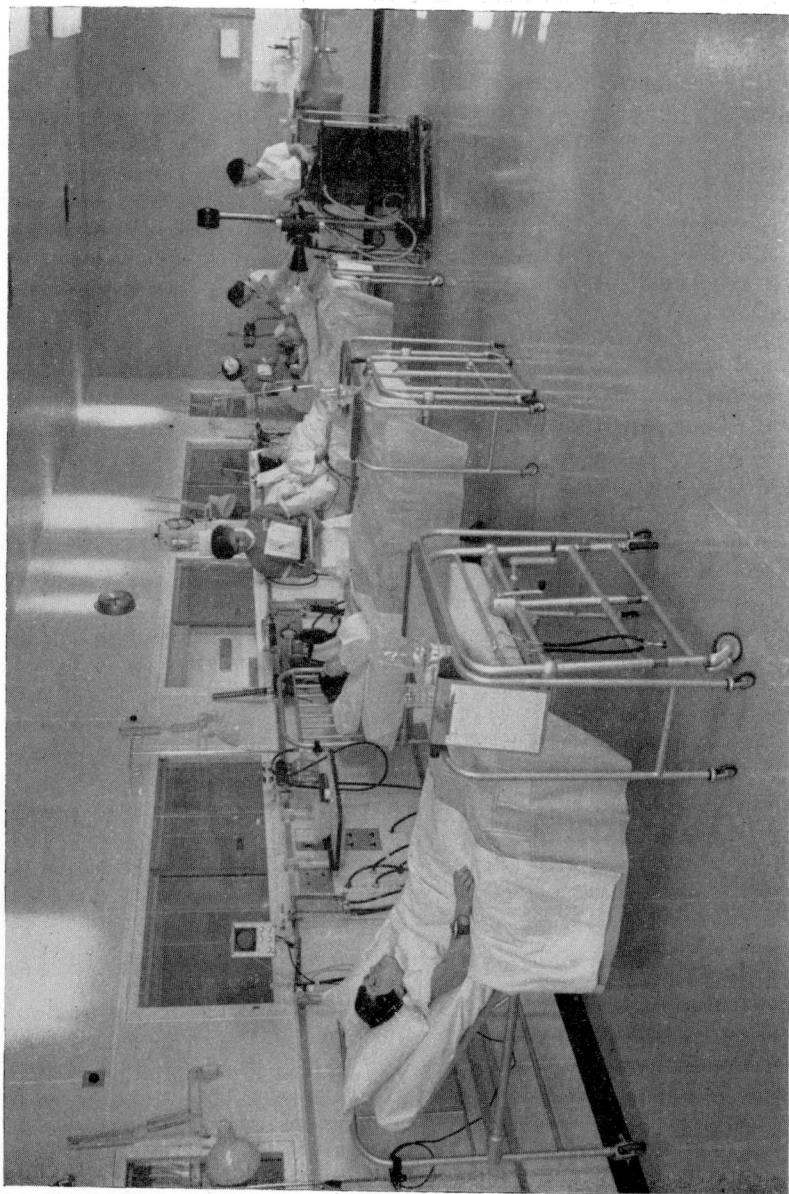

3.—An Open Ward.

majority of patients were confined to bed, and one bathroom and two lavatories were considered adequate for 25 patients. Today, however, the situation is quite different and most patients get up for part of the day. Modern hospital planning allows for this, with good toilet facilities and sitting or "day" rooms for these patients. Also the tendency is for smaller units —i.e. 2, 4 or 6 beds being grouped together. This makes it easier for patients to have more privacy; in open wards this is achieved by the use of individual bed curtains.

NURSE TRAINING

The concept of nurse training and the employment of professional nurses were not thought of before the 19th century. Prior to this most nursing had been done in the home by friends and relatives, or in hospital by the Religious Sisters, or by untrained women mostly from the domestic servant class. These women were poorly paid, worked under appalling conditions in many cases, and did little that would nowadays be regarded as "nursing". Sisters and matrons were often drawn from a rather higher class, but were responsible in the main only for domestic and household management. Although no formal training was given, it is probable that many learned from the doctors under whom they worked, and that some of them did their work well. Others, however, did not, and drunkenness, pilfering from patients and immorality were fairly common. Some of the worst conditions existed in the workhouses where those paupers who were well were made to look after those who were sick, with appalling results.

In the United States conditions were not much better, and in Bellevue Hospital, New York, nurses were drawn from the inmates of the nearby prison. On the Continent, the greater numbers of Religious Sisters raised the standard of care to some extent, but conditions were still bad, and in the Hôtel-Dieu in Paris it was common to find 5, 6 or 7 patients to a bed.

Reform came in the middle of the 19th century and with it the idea of some training for nurses; it coincided, in this country at any rate, with the growing desire on the part of young women to have some suitable occupation outside the home. Many of the early reformers still linked the idea of nursing with a religious order; in 1836, Pastor Theodore Fliedner. who had already done much work among discharged prisoners in Germany, revived the Church Order of Deaconesses in Kaiserswerth; the deaconesses received a brief training and then went out to nurse, under supervision, in nearby hospitals. The work grew rapidly and soon spread beyond the borders of Germany, deaconesses being sent to the U.S.A., the Middle East and to London, where they staffed the German Hospital and what is now the Prince of Wales Hospital, Tottenham. By 1900 there were some 35,000 deaconesses working all over the world.

In England a Church of England Sisterhood was founded in 1848—St. John's House, Fitzroy Square. Here young women were admitted at 18 years of age and paid for a two-year training which they received at either the Westminster or the Middlesex Hospitals; the work expanded and later the nurses took over the whole of the staffing of King's College Hospital. A similar organisation was All Saints Sisterhood which became responsible for staffing University College Hospital. Nurses who worked for the Sisterhoods received board and lodging and a very small salary. It is interesting to note that Sisters were still recruited separately, had a shorter training and more freedom.

The first real attempt to separate nursing from the religious "motherhouses" was in Switzerland. In 1859 Comtesse de Gasparin started a school of nursing in Lausanne—La Source. She felt strongly that nurses should be paid sufficient salary to be independent of any organisation, and that the individual should be completely free and not bound by vows. She also believed that devotion was not enough and that a thorough training was necessary. She finally endowed the school, so safeguarding it from financial difficulties. She was closely followed by Florence Nightingale who, in 1860, founded and endowed the Nightingale School.

The Crimean War had showed the public in Britain the inadequacy of the nursing service. The French and British were fighting alongside the Turks against Russia, and as casualties mounted news began to reach home of the appalling conditions in the hospitals; the French wounded were cared for by the Sisters of Charity, but there was no one to look after the British wounded. The Secretary at War, Sidney Herbert, wrote to Florence Nightingale who had offered her services, asking her to organise and superintend a group of women nurses to go to the Crimea. She already had a great interest in, and knowledge of, nursing; she had visited hospitals in different parts of Europe, and had spent time at Kaiserswerth, and with the Sisters of Charity in Paris. In England she had been superintendent of a nursing home in Harley Street, and had worked at the Middlesex Hospital. She also had a very influential social position.

The recruitment of suitable nurses proved extraordinarily difficult, since so few were available. Eventually 38 were chosen —to nurse all the wounded in the British Army—from Roman Catholic and Anglican Sisterhoods, St. John's House and various hospitals. With Miss Nightingale in charge the party set off. The story of the conditions they found, the opposition of the Army and the work that was done is too well known to be repeated here; however, as a result the public became aware of the great need for nursing reform, and as an expression of gratitude to Miss Nightingale, the *Nightingale Fund* was set up and £44,000 collected, £9,000 being subscribed by the Army (1855).

The Fund was used to set up and endow a training school where nurses could receive the type of training Miss Nightingale felt they needed; she chose St. Thomas's Hospital, because it was about to be rebuilt and had as Matron a woman whom she felt to be eminently suitable—Mrs. Wardroper. The original course of training at the Nightingale School was for a period of one year. Probationers were carefully selected by Mrs. Wardroper and Miss Nightingale, who placed more emphasis on character than on education. They had to "live in" in a nurses' home, were given board and lodging free and a sum of £10 for the course. They were supervised closely both in the wards and off duty. After a few years a second course was started for lady pupils who paid for their board and lodging during training. Other hospitals followed the Nightingale School and started training schemes of their own, and many of the lady pupils, on completing their course at St. Thomas's, went on to become matrons of hospitals all over Britain. The idea of a woman exercising power and being head of the nursing service was absolutely new and was resented in many cases by the medical staff and the hospital administrators. However, Miss Nightingale's influence was great, and she backed her trainees whenever possible. Gradually the new ideas began to take hold; some were quite popular, particularly the training of lady pupils, who, in many cases, paid quite a large premium for their training. Improvements in the care of patients became obvious and in the public mind nursing became not only respectable but a vocation. The Nightingale system spread not only to the voluntary hospitals, but to the Poor Law Institutions as well. It was based on the position of the Matron, who was solely responsible for the nursing staff as well as for the domestic service, the system of "living in" for probationers who were responsible to a home sister and whose free time was to some extent controlled, and the theoretical and practical instruction of the nurses in training who were taught and supervised in the wards by the ward sister.

By 1900 nursing was popular as a vocation for women and the demand for their services was increasing. The standards of training varied widely from hospital to hospital, as did its length. Each hospital issued its own certificate to those who had satisfactorily completed training, but many felt that some central organisation should exist to set a standard and keep a register of trained nurses. The most militant supporter of this view was Mrs. Bedford Fenwick, who was appointed Matron of St. Bartholomew's Hospital in 1881, at the age of 24, but who left active nursing for marriage in 1887. With her husband she campaigned vigorously for educational standards for entry to training schools, more theoretical instruction, a qualifying examination for which nurses must pay a fee and a national register. Miss Nightingale did not agree; she felt that character was as important as education and that neither this nor the ability to be a good nurse could be tested by an examination; also that a national standard and register would invariably lower the high standards achieved by many training schools. For these reasons she opposed the whole idea and such was her influence that the dispute over registration continued for many years after her death.

Every year from 1904 to 1914, Bills to introduce registration for nurses were laid before Parliament; there were by now many organisations representing different sections of the profession, but as they were unable to agree on what they wanted and as there was still strong opposition to registration, no Bill was passed. With the outbreak of the First World War the dispute faded into the background.

As had happened during the Crimean War, the need for nurses was felt acutely, public admiration was aroused for their work, and some of the weaknesses and discrepancies in existing training schemes were brought to light. By the end of the war the nurses themselves were far more outspoken in their wish for registration—influenced perhaps by the fear of the large numbers of "untrained" women who had been working in hospitals during the war; also they now had the vote. A new professional organisation—the College of Nursing—had come into being in 1916 and was becoming powerful. Finally, in 1919, a Bill was introduced which gave the Minister of Health power to appoint the first General Nursing Council, which was to be the statutory body responsible for nurse training and the registration of nurses.

The story of the first General Nursing Council and the battles which ensued before it was decided which "trained" nurses might have their names entered on the Register makes fascinating reading. Mrs. Bedford Fenwick—now over 60—was a most voluble member of the first Council. Applications from practising nurses were received and considered until 1923, and at the same time the Council drew up a syllabus of training which they hoped would be compulsory; however, the Minister of Health would only allow it to be issued as a guide to hospitals, since he feared that a strict syllabus would increase the shortage of nurses. In 1925 the first examination was held and for the first time nurses became State Registered as the result of an examination; the pattern for modern conditions of training was set.

Today the statutory bodies controlling nurse training are the General Nursing Councils for England and Wales, Scotland, and Northern Ireland. The Council for England and Wales has 36 members (this number will rise to 40 in 1970), half appointed by the Minister of Health and others, and half elected by Registered Nurses. In 1970 22 members will be elected and 18 appointed by the Secretary of State for Health.

Its functions include:

1. The inspection and approval of hospitals as nurse training schools.

2. The organisation of qualifying examinations.
3. The maintenance of Registers of Nurses who are successful in these examinations.

The Registers which are maintained are:

1. For general trained nurses and   S.R.N.
   For nurses trained in the care of:
2. The mentally ill   R.M.N.
3. Sick children   R.S.C.N.
4. The mentally subnormal   R.N.M.S.

All are three-year trainings; since 1965 students have no longer been accepted for fever training, since the decline in the incidence of infectious diseases has limited the experience available. This type of experience will be available to some nurses in general training as one of their two specialities and hospitals with large units for such diseases as poliomyelitis will continue to organise their own post-registration courses.

The full Council meets on the fourth Friday of alternate months and the general public may attend the meetings; much of the work is done by various sub-committees. An annual Report is made to the Secretary of State and copies are available.

Training Schools.—At present the age of entry for nurse training is 18 and the minimum age of registration is 21.

Training Schools for nurses have an Introductory Course lasting 8 weeks in many cases. During this time classes are given in anatomy and physiology and other subjects, but the main emphasis is on basic nursing and an introduction to hospital life. Vistis are made to the wards and departments and other places of interest; a programme is arranged so that each student works for short periods under supervision in the ward to which she will be allocated at the end of the introductory period. Most of the tuition is given by qualified nurse tutors. The Introductory Course is intended to help the student to adapt to her new environment and to equip her with skills she will need during the early months of training so that, on its completion, the first full day in the ward is a happy occasion for which she is adequately prepared.

The student nurse returns to the School for periods of study at intervals throughout her training, in order that she may be given the necessary theoretical background to enable her to nurse her patients intelligently. Most hospitals use the "block" system, which means that nurses leave the wards for a "block" of several weeks each year. During this time they are freed from the responsibility of patient care and are able to concentrate on, enjoy and benefit from this period of study. Another system is the "study day"; here the student nurse spends one full day each week in the School for about six months of each year. With either system, lectures are given by physicians, surgeons, tutors, ward sisters and many others. In addition, tuition is given in the wards, between periods of study, by ward sisters, tutors or clinical teachers.

The State Enrolled Nurse.—For those who desire a shorter training with less emphasis on theory, a 2-year course is available leading to State Enrolment (S.E.N.). The age of entry is as for the 3 year training: the pupil nurse starts her training with a 4-week introductory period: the remainder of the 2 years is spent in the wards or departments, and theoretical instruction is given in weekly study half-days or in regular blocks of 1 week duration. During the second year an assessment is carried out by General Nursing Council assessors and if this is satisfactory, the pupil then completes her training and becomes enrolled.

Many hospitals of all types offer training for both the Register and Roll and it is hoped that the number of State Enrolled Nurses will continue to increase. This form of training is eminently suitable for those more interested in continuing patient care than in further academic training leading to administrative or teaching positions.

A number of hospitals are now giving various experimental types of training which are designed for those with specific abilities or interests.

References and suggestions for further reading

ABEL-SMITH, B. (1960). *A History of the Nursing Profession.* (London, William Heinemann, Ltd.)

SEYMER, L. R. (1957). *A General History of Nursing*, 4th ed. (London, Faber & Faber, Ltd.)

BENDALL and RAYBOULD. *A History of the General Nursing Council* (1969) (London, H. K. Lewis & Co. Ltd.)

Chapter II

THE HEALTHY PERSON

GROWTH AND DEVELOPMENT

Foundations of health are laid before a baby is actually born. Factors affecting the growth and development of the foetus are the general health and well-being of the mother including freedom from infection, and her nutrition during pregnancy. In this country many facilities are available for good ante-natal care and safe delivery of the baby. Once born, his development is influenced to a large extent by his environment.

During the first year of life a baby needs food, warmth and fresh air, a feeling of security, and an opportunity to develop simple muscular skills.

In the early days milk is the staple food; the age of weaning varies, but 3 to 4 months is a common time to introduce solids. By the age of 9 to 10 months the timing and content of meals should coincide with those of the rest of the family, allowance being made for the presence or absence of teeth!

Light warm clothing which does not hamper movement is desirable; it must be remembered that a baby feels changes in temperature more than an adult, and is very susceptible to extremes. Some period of each day should be spent in the fresh air if possible.

Newborn babies have fears, just like the rest of us. They are upset by inexpert handling, sudden noise and a feeling of restriction of movement. At this stage there is little awareness of personalities and so little fear of strangers.

The term *milestones* is used to describe certain activities reached by a certain age. It is essential to remember that there is a wide difference between individual babies, and much unhappiness is caused by comparisons either within or outside the family. However, at 6 months many babies are sitting unsupported, cutting their first teeth and beginning to grasp objects. At 1 year crawling is well established, recognition of familiar faces and voices is obvious, sounds are being made and some words have meaning for the child. He is no longer a baby and will soon be a toddler.

From 18 months to about 3 years of age is often a difficult time for both the child and his parents. He is extremely active, easily bored, very possessive, especially where his mother is concerned, completely unreasonable at times and utterly unsociable as regards other children. At his best he is quite adorable, at his most difficult he brings out the worst in those around him. In most families three things cause difficulty and worry—toilet training, meals and sleep. The golden rule is to avoid direct battle, and appear to be as little emotionally involved as possible. The most effective way of dealing with complete refusal, or temper, is to provide an alternative interest, and the problem is soon forgotten (by the child). For guidance in this matter, the nurse cannot do better than to read *Do babies have worries*, published by the National Association for Mental Health.

At about the age of $3\frac{1}{2}$ a happier phase begins. The child becomes much more co-operative, sociable and anxious to please, and can now perform simple tasks for himself. He likes the company of other children and is happy away from his mother for longer periods. Two attributes of this age group are unending questions and an extremely vivid imagination. Independence must be encouraged before school age is reached.

At 5 years old (in this country) the child's formal education begins, and his horizon widens. Over the next few years he becomes less and less obviously dependent on home and family as skills and interests develop, but his need for understanding and security remain. Group friendships and "gang" activities are increasingly important, and boys and girls develop different interests, and have little time for each other. Parents are wise to provide increasing opportunities for responsibility and independence.

The next major event for most children is a change of school at the age of 11. This precedes the gradual transition from child to adolescent.

The period known as adolescence brings changes, and with them many problems. For the girl it means the onset of menstruation, and physical development occurs, including enlargement of the breasts. Reassurance and help is often necessary at this stage, particularly as regards personal hygiene and activities during her periods. The phrase "not well" is unfortunate

16

—menstruation is a normal process and should not interfere with normal life in any way. Discomfort or pain associated with menstruation is quite common, especially during the "teens", but it is rarely severe enough to incapacitate.

For the boy there are also bodily changes, including enlargement of the sex organs and "breaking" of the voice. These changes occur 1 to 2 years later than in those described for girls.

For both, physical development is often faster than muscular co-ordination and this may lead to clumsiness. In addition, acne (blackheads or spots) may cause considerable embarrassment. Although it is little consolation at the time, this is merely a phase, and will pass.

Emotional changes also take place; these show themselves in many ways, and account in part for the so-called "difficult teenager". Boys and girls begin to take a greater interest in their appearance and in each other, and go through a period of experimenting with dress, hair styles and make-up. For the first time, money, a career and the need for social acceptance become important, and although it is not obvious, much support and encouragement is needed from parents and older friends.

Work is very important and it is necessary to choose the right career early in life if adulthood and the later years are to be happy (and healthy). The years between 21 and 45 are those when an individual is at the height of his powers and physical, emotional and intellectual maturity are achieved. Twenty-one is the accepted "coming of age" but maturity is difficult to define and is reached at varying ages. The mature person is able to enjoy life fully and to deal confidently with problems as they arise. For most people adulthood brings marriage and a family, and thus increasing responsibilities. Many devote time and energy to help others in their community by accepting civic duties.

From 45 to 65 responsibilities are probably fewer, children grow up and leave home and it is necessary to make adjustments. There is a gradual decline of physical and mental powers which is compensated for by an increase in judgment due to experience.

For women, middle age means the cessation of menstruation which may be accompanied by emotional difficulties, mild depression being common. However, the majority adjust well and approach old age (senescence) and retirement sensibly.

More people today reach old age than ever before: in 1970 17% of the population will be over 65.

The official age of retirement in this country is 60 to 65, although many people continue working beyond this age. Preparations are necessary for a happy retirement as surveys have shown that rapid deterioration in physical and mental capacity are common in those who have no interests outside their work. Old people value their independence. An active mind and a healthy body, combined with the company of their family and friends, are essential if this independence is to be maintained.

One of the great problems of our time is the increasing number of lonely old people. A tendency has been to group old people together; a happier solution, now being realised, is to provide housing and other amenities within the community at large.

PHYSICAL NEEDS

In order to live, the following are necessary:

1. Food and drink   2. Fresh air
3. Shelter   4. Rest and sleep

Variations in health occur if these are inadequate.

1. Food and drink.—Although the total amount of food available is probably sufficient for the world's needs, mal-distribution and under-development lead to great differences in standards of living. It is estimated that one-half of the population of the world is undernourished. Conversely, some countries have more food than is needed, and, in fact, in the so-called civilised communities, overeating contributes to much ill-health. In this country, standards are high, and with full employment deficiency diseases are rare. In addition, certain age groups benefit from cheap or free supplements.

- (a) **Children under five.**—Cheap milk is provided; for infants this may be in the form of dried milk. Concentrated fruit juices and cod-liver oil are also available.
- (b) **School children.**—All children at maintained Primary and Special schools and junior pupils at all age schools have $\frac{1}{3}$ pint of milk a day, free of charge, during the morning break, and may also have their midday meal at school at a subsidised rate.

18

(c) **Pregnant and nursing mothers.**—These women receive vitamin supplements and some milk at special prices.

(d) **Old people.**—Although the aged are not automatically provided for, in many towns voluntary services, in collaboration with local health authorities, organise a "Meals on Wheels" service whereby a hot meal is delivered several times a week. The Department of Social Security will also help those unable to provide for themselves, either by supplementing their pensions or by supplying food.

2. **Fresh air** would appear to be available for everyone; but in this respect the highly developed countries suffer most. In many towns, especially in industrial areas, the air is grossly polluted by smoke from domestic chimneys, factories and most forms of transport. In the winter months there is the additional hazard of fog, or "smog", which is a mixture of smoke and moisture, highly lethal to the elderly and to sufferers from chronic chest conditions.

Following a particularly severe episode in 1952, the Government brought in the Clean Air Act, under which many towns and cities have instituted smokeless zones. In these areas it is an offence to burn fuels which produce smoke, and this has led to a change in traditional methods of heating.

3. **Shelter.**—With regard to shelter, housing is a major problem in this country. Many houses are old, lacking in modern conveniences and overcrowded in some areas. The cost of land and building is high, and at present the number of houses being completed is far too small to accommodate all those who are looking for homes. Few people are actually homeless, but many need rehousing. Where possible the tendency is to rehouse families either in multi-storey flats, or on new housing estates. These are modern in design, and are often planned to include garden spaces, wide roads, recreational facilities and shops. The provision of "Green Belt" areas has added to amenities and controlled the "mushroom" growth of new towns. While this is admirable, and beneficial to health in many respects, it has had the effect of breaking family ties, and separating close-knit communities. In many instances, rehousing has meant a

move of several miles, necessitating new jobs, new schools and the need to make new friends and acquire new interests. For many who have grown up with numerous relatives and friends nearby to call on when the occasion arises, it has been difficult to adjust to a new and strange community. In short, the material needs have been met but the result has been an increase in problems of loneliness and insecurity.

4. **Rest and sleep.**—The amount of rest and sleep required varies according to age. The newborn baby sleeps for about 20 hours out of 24. At 2 years most children sleep for 12 hours at night, and have a rest during the afternoon. By the age of 10, 9 to 10 hours is sufficient, and most adults sleep from 6 to 8 hours.

With advancing age the need for sleep lessens, but it will be noted that although their nights may be short and disturbed, old people tend to doze at intervals during the day.

With the increasing pace of modern life, periods of recreation are important. Many of today's illnesses belong to the group termed "stress disorders", and are directly related to a failure to obtain adequate physical, mental and emotional rest.

MENTAL HEALTH AND EFFECT OF ENVIRONMENT

The World Health Organisation defines health as "a state of physical, mental and social well-being and not merely the absence of disease".

These three react on each other and cannot be separated. Mental health shows in the way an individual adapts and reacts to situations and people around him. Most people have occasional difficulty in adjusting to their problems, but providing adjustment is made without too much emotional trauma, this cannot be termed ill-health. However, for some, continual stress may be a predisposing factor to illness.

The pressure of life today has increased the stresses under which we live. Since the last war, standards of living have risen and articles formally classed as luxuries are now considered necessities; this has produced the unending battle to "keep up with the Joneses". In many cases it has also led to young wives and mothers going out to work to supplement the family income. Although satisfactory arrangements can be made for their children, the result may be to deprive the young ones of one of their deepest needs—a happy, secure home.

Early selection for different types of secondary schooling has now been virtually abandoned in this country: however, examination pressures remain and can still cause considerable stress if parents expect too much of children or give the impression that their future is dependent on examination results.

The adolescent, today, has more money and more freedom than at any time before. He is also brought up in a world with rapidly changing moral values; all this may produce problems which are beyond his experience and his degree of emotional development.

People of all ages are spending increasing amounts of money on pep-pills to boost their morale and tranquillisers to calm them down.

It is a sad reflection of our time that many of the hospital beds in this country are used for the treatment of patients who have failed to adjust and are, in some degree, mentally ill.

Mental health is a precious thing; one parent has stated that his aim for his child is that he should be: "a newer kind of human being; an aware person, without fear and with love; a sound individual, adequate to live anywhere on earth and loving life everywhere and always". (*Death be not Proud*, John Gunther, N.Y., 1949.)

The environment can be thought of as the total situation in which a person lives, works and plays—and several factors have already been mentioned. It will to a certain extent mould the character and personality, and affect health.

Obviously life in the country has certain advantages over life in an industrial town, in that the tempo is slower and the air fresher. Equally, whether in town or country, living space and amenities available are important; in a large family many activities are in progress at the same time; this can cause friction if space is limited.

An interesting job is essential, since boredom, frustration and lack of incentive can undermine health and increase minor ailments. Occupational hazards are not always apparent. For example, the sedentary worker is prone to certain disorders in that he does not take enough exercise, while the miner, though active, is at risk through inhaling coal dust. In the last few

21

years occupational health has become an important branch of medicine.

Included in the environment must be the people with whom we live and work. The phrase "human relationships" is a new description of the old problem of getting on with each other. Many of the day-to-day irritations can be traced to a lack of understanding, and a breakdown in communications.

Thus, in nursing, the ability to like people, to accept them for what they are, and to have some understanding of their problems, is of fundamental importance. It is possible to become a State Registered Nurse by assimilating theoretical knowledge and acquiring technical skills; but to be a good nurse requires much more than this. For a time, at least, she is an essential part of her patients' environment.

THE INCIDENCE OF DISEASE

One of the greatest advances in medicine in the last 50 years has been the decline in the incidence of infectious disease in this country. This is due to many factors, including:

(*a*) A general rise in the standards of living.

(*b*) The introduction of large-scale immunisation programmes.

(*c*) The development of the antibiotic drugs.

(*a*) The rise in the standard of living, particularly with regard to housing and nutrition, has already been referred to.

(*b*) The immunisation programmes are the responsibility of local health authorities and general practitioners. At present vaccination and immunisation are available against the following diseases:

Diphtheria ⎫
Whooping-cough ⎬ often given together as the
Tetanus ⎭   triple vaccine
Smallpox
Poliomyelitis
Tuberculosis
Measles

In some areas a quadruple vaccine is available, combining

the poliomyelitis vaccine with the triple vaccine.

Perhaps one of the most striking results of mass immunisation has been the virtual eradication of diphtheria, which 30 years ago killed several thousand people each year. Unfortunately, because of this, the rate of immunisation has declined and so, should an epidemic occur, large sections of the community would be at risk. A similar decline in the vaccination rate was illustrated during the smallpox outbreak of 1962.

(c) The antibiotic drugs, of which penicillin is the best known, have been produced on a large scale since the war. They have completely altered the course and treatment of many infections, but as yet none has been found to have much effect on the smallest organisms, the viruses.

On the whole, the health of the nation is better than at any previous time in our history. The infant mortality rate is at its lowest, and children of all ages are taller and heavier than those of 30 years ago. Many diseases can now be prevented and many others diagnosed early enough to be successfully treated; men and women are living longer, the life expectancy for a man being 69 years and for a woman 74 years.

In spite of this, certain trends give rise to anxiety. For example, at least 15 people die on the roads each day, and 20 as a result of accidents in their homes; in addition, thousands are injured, many seriously. The vast majority of these accidents are preventable. On the roads, all age groups are at risk, but in the home the very young and the elderly are the most accident prone.

There is an increase in the incidence of certain types of malignant disease, particularly lung cancer, and also, as has been mentioned, in stress disorders and mental illness.

It may seem strange that, in these circumstances, plans are being made to reduce the number of beds available for the treatment of patients with mental disorders. In fact many can now be treated as out-patients, or in psychiatric units in general hospitals.

These and other trends are reflected in hospital planning, e.g.

(i) an increase in the number of maternity beds to cope with the preference for having a baby in hospital;

(ii) an emphasis on the provision of Regional Accident Centres;

(iii) the closing of many infectious disease hospitals and sanatoria.

(iv) the provision of all types of hospital service in one unit—the new district general hospital.

(v) an emphasis on the need to improve facilities for the mentally subnormal.

Chapter III

ADMISSION TO HOSPITAL

Although a healthy community is desirable, everyone becomes ill at some time during their life. In most cases the sick are cared for at home, by doctors, nurses, relatives or neighbours. It is estimated, however, that, on average, people are admitted to hospital for some reason or other, on five occasions during their lifetime.

People come to a hospital ward either in an emergency or as an arranged admission. It is desirable to consider these separately as the circumstances and problems involved are rather different; in both cases the nurse should remember that the patient's first impressions are of great importance.

ARRANGED ADMISSION

These patients—sometimes described as "list" or "cold" cases—are already known to the hospital and will have attended the out-patients department on one or several occasions. They are sent to a specialist clinic, either by their general practitioner, by an industrial medical officer or, in the case of a child, they may be referred by the School Health Service. At the clinic they are examined, a history is taken and any necessary investigations carried out. In some cases admission is recommended and the patient's name is added to a waiting list. In due course, when a bed becomes vacant in the appropriate ward, a letter is sent advising the patient of the date when he is to come in; many hospitals also enclose useful information in the form of a pamphlet, giving such details as general ward routine, shopping facilities available and visiting hours. The letter will give the name of the ward and the time when he should arrive—usually mid-morning or afternoon.

The time between attendance at the out-patients clinic and the date of admission gives the patient ample opportunity to adjust to the idea that he needs hospital care and to make any necessary arrangements. It is unfortunate that in some cases, owing to shortage of beds, many months may elapse before treatment is available.

When the day arrives, the patient presents himself at the reception desk of the hospital and is usually directed straight to the ward. He brings with him such articles as pyjamas, soap, notepaper and any personal items listed in the pamphlet or hospital letter. He is usually accompanied by a relative or friend.

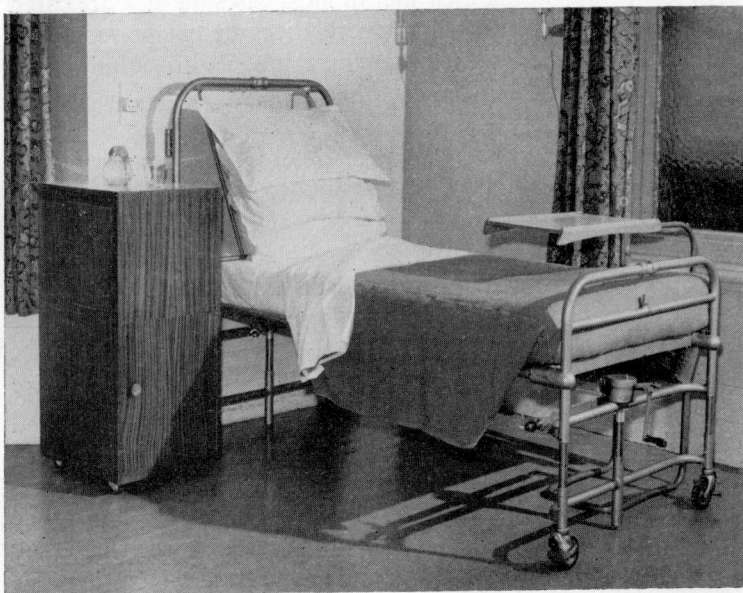

FIG. 4.—Admission Bed.

Although he may be apprehensive, the patient has some idea of his illness and his probable length of stay in hospital, and he will have met at least one of the doctors who will be caring for him. In the ward his records will be available from the out-patient department, this is useful as he can be greeted by name and will feel that he is expected.

Preparations for his arrival include seeing that a bed and locker are ready for him, preferably near to someone about his own age.

Methods of bedmaking vary from hospital to hospital—in most cases this empty bed will be made in the same way as at home.

Many of our hospitals are old and have little storage space

for patients' clothes. For this reason—and also because he is likely to be examined by a doctor later in the day—the patient is asked to undress, either at his bedside with the curtains drawn, or in the bathroom. The clothes can then be taken home. Any clothes kept in the ward must be listed in the appropriate book, checked by the nurse and put away safely. It is unnecessary in most cases to ask the patient to bath at this point; the majority of people, wishing to appear at their best, will have made certain that they are clean before setting out. It is equally unnecessary to ask the patient to get into bed, unless his doctor is in the ward and ready to examine him. It must be remembered that these patients are not acutely ill, and have probably been following their normal occupation until the previous day.

The nurse should explain the ward geography—particularly the whereabouts of the toilets; she can introduce the newcomer to his immediate neighbours and clarify any points that may be worrying him. The friends or relatives should be allowed into the ward to see him before going home. Visiting cards—if used —are issued and the hospital phone number and ward extension given. It is advisable at this time to check the patient's records, in case any details have changed, and to make sure that a phone number is available where his relatives can be reached, or a message left.

Once the visitors have left, points such as mealtimes—which often differ from those at home—should be explained to the patient; various uniforms and their meanings are of interest too. Routine tests such as temperature, pulse and respiration rates and ward urine tests are often left till later.

EMERGENCY ADMISSION

An increasing number of people come to hospital as a result of accidents or sudden illness. It is reasonable to assume that these patients are acutely ill, and in need of urgent care and attention.

They come to the casualty department—usually by ambulance; occasionally they arrive on foot. Their arrival is unexpected and in many cases the hospital knows nothing of them or their previous history. For the patient there are problems apart from his condition; he is mentally unprepared for admission to hospital and has had no time to put his affairs in order. He is often unaccompanied, has brought nothing with him and may have little idea of what is wrong with him. Obviously, these emergencies may occur at any time during the 24 hours, and may present problems as far as empty beds are concerned —especially during the winter months.

The patient is examined in the casualty department and, if possible, details and a history are obtained. The ward is notified of the impending admission and details of his condition are given so that suitable arrangements can be made.

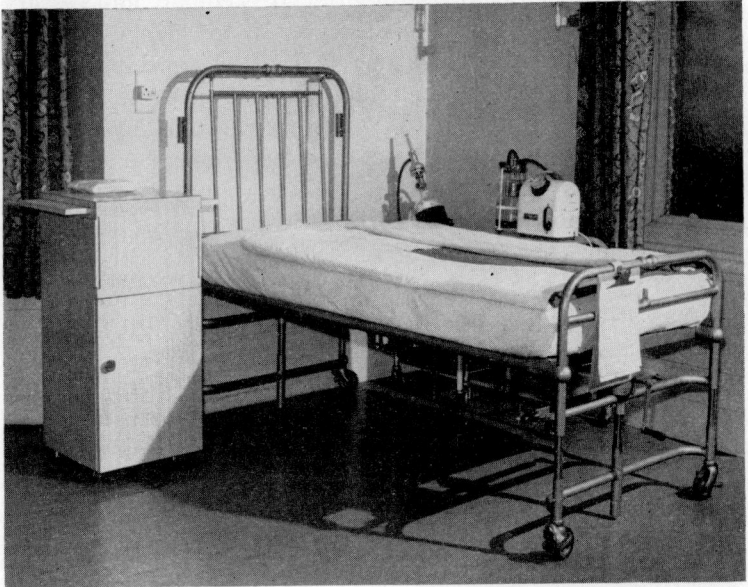

FIG. 5.—Emergency Admission Bed.

The preparations include—first the bed; this is made so that it is suitable for someone who will be confined to bed; a waterproof cover is placed under the bottom sheet, unless there is one on the mattress. In some hospitals extra protection is provided in the form of a "draw" sheet. This is a narrow sheet placed across the middle of the bed; the term "draw" sheet is an old one, derived from the fact that the sheet should be long enough to be drawn through if the patient becomes hot or uncomfortable. The top bedclothes are not tucked in, but folded back to form a pack which can be lifted clear of the bed; this is necessary as the patient may arrive on a stretcher and have to be lifted on to the bed.

If pillows are allowed these may, in certain cases, be protected by waterproof covers under the cotton pillow-cases. Occasionally the bed may be warmed by the inclusion of hot-water bottles or electric blankets, but these are removed before the patient is put into bed. If possible the bed is moved to a quiet corner of the ward, near to sister's desk or office; if the emergency occurs at night, it is preferable to admit the patient to a side ward—this prevents too much disturbance for the other patients.

Articles of clothing, such as pyjamas, must be at hand, and soap, towels and flannels placed in the locker. Various charts are collected, e.g. treatment, diet, temperature, pulse and respiration, and any others which may be applicable to the particular patient. Other apparatus—such as oxygen equipment and suction apparatus—may be needed.

When the patient arrives in the ward, he is lifted gently into bed and the top bedclothes placed over him and tucked in in the usual way; if he is still fully clothed, he is undressed and put into night clothes. Should a relative be present she should be reassured and seated comfortably in a nearby waiting-room or office. A cup of tea is often appreciated and an assurance can be given that the doctor or sister will see her when the patient has been made comfortable. If no relatives are present, it is the hospital's responsibility to inform them of the patient's admission.

The patient, meanwhile, is seen by the ward doctor, and any immediate treatment ordered and carried out. His position in bed will depend on the nature of his illness—for example, a patient with pneumonia will be more comfortable sitting up. In the majority of cases the patient's first need is rest, and he should be disturbed as little as possible.

He may need bathing in bed at some stage, but this can usually wait till he has rested and his condition improved. Before giving a drink the nurse must check with sister or the senior nurse that the patient is allowed fluids by mouth; she should also remember that the patient may wish to pass urine and offer a bedpan or urinal. The first specimen of urine passed should be saved for ward testing. Temperature, pulse and respiration rates are taken and recorded on the chart. Explanations, such as those given to patients admitted from the waiting list, can often wait, but any immediate problems that are worrying him must be dealt with. As soon as possible the relatives are seen, and the patient's condition explained to them. Any information not so far obtained can be got from them; this should include the patient's full name, address, age, next-of-kin, occupation, religion and private doctor, also the relative's telephone number. If the patient's condition is critical they may be asked to stay, or told that they can visit or telephone at any time. The clothes are handed to them, together with any valuables. If possible they should be allowed to see the patient before leaving. If no relatives are present, any valuables are listed, checked and locked in the hospital safe.

Social and financial difficulties often occur, following an emergency admission; the medical-social worker, if notified, can help with these.

THE HOSPITAL WARD

In many general hospitals a ward contains 20 to 30 beds; the patients in these beds may be either arranged admissions, or emergency cases.

Just as at home, a ward needs adequate lighting, an efficient heating system and some form of ventilation.

Lighting.—During the daytime, natural lighting is often adequate; this is helped if wall surfaces are clean and light in colour. Artificial lights may be divided into three groups: first, the main ward lights, which also incorporate "night" lights; secondly, individual lights; and thirdly, portable lights of various kinds.

1. *The main ward lights* are set high in the ceiling, have globe shades to prevent glare and are controlled by "two-way" switches; when the patients have been tucked down for the night the lights are lowered to a faint glow—not enough to keep the patients awake, but sufficient to allow movement and observation by the night staff.

2. *Individual lights* are situated over each bed, and at other strategic points, such as sister's desk. They are shaded to direct the beam of light downwards, so that the patient can read or write in comfort, and also receive attention at night without disturbing the patient in the next bed.

3. *Portable lamps* vary in type and are used to provide light for

detailed examination and treatment, electric points being available at various places round the ward.

Heating.—The majority of hospitals and wards are now centrally heated; heating is provided by steam or hot water circulating in radiators or wall panels. A suitable temperature for an open ward is 18° C. (65° F.). This can be controlled by turning radiators on or off, and by opening or shutting windows. Side wards may have additional heating in the form of electric fires. It must be remembered that a comfortable temperature for nurses working in the wards may not necessarily be adequate for a patient lying still in bed or sitting in a chair; bed-jackets and extra blankets should be given, or removed, as desired.

Ventilation.—In this country, owing to inadequately heated homes, many people object to open windows. In hospital, however, good ventilation is necessary to prevent the ward becoming stuffy and to lessen the risk of cross-infection. Direct draughts should be avoided by careful spacing of open windows.

NOISE IN HOSPITALS

Noise is a modern problem in hospital and much has been written on this subject. It seems that sudden, unexpected noise is more distressing to the sick than everyday sounds to which they are accustomed, such as vacuum cleaners and washing up.

The introduction of "disposable" equipment and the general use of plastics may reduce the amount of noise; but nurses have a responsibility to do all they can to lessen this problem. Hospital planners can assist with the introduction of such equipment as acoustic tiling or double glazing; but all those who come to the wards in any capacity must remember that the clatter of leather sole shoes or the noise made by loose fitting "casuals" or slippers, are among the things most often mentioned by tired patients.

One hundred years ago, Florence Nightingale wrote: "Unnecessary noise is the most cruel absence of care which can be inflicted on sick or well", and the same is true today.

EQUIPMENT

To many new student nurses a ward contains several mysterious and often unidentifiable things; in fact, much of the equipment and materials used are similar to those found in everyday life.

31

The beds are usually higher, and commonly have a metal frame; the height makes nursing care easier, but can be a disadvantage to frail or elderly patients when getting in or out; the frames are easier to keep clean than wooden or upholstered bases. Many firms now make beds which can be raised or lowered when necessary.

The mattress, sheets, blankets, bedcovers, pillows and pillowcases are the same as those used at home, although a modern tendency is to use cotton cellular blankets as these are easier to launder than wool. Flannelette sheets may be used for extra warmth.

CARE OF EQUIPMENT

Linen.—This is changed as necessary, dirty linen being sent to the laundry in bags. These bags are fixed to a movable stand —or linen carrier—which can be taken round when beds are being made. Linen soiled by excreta is usually collected separately and the container marked before being sent to the laundry. Torn or stained linen is not used; it is set aside for replacement or repair.

Blankets.—As mentioned, cotton cellular blankets are now in common use. These should be sent to the laundry when soiled, or when a patient goes home. Special blankets—often coloured—may be used in the casualty or other departments of the hospital.

Rubber articles.—These should be stored in a cool dry place, and not folded, articles such as hot-water bottles and rubber rings being slightly inflated. After use they may be washed in warm soapy water and powdered if necessary. In most hospitals thin polythene sheeting has taken the place of rubber mackintoshes. This is cheaper and is thrown away after use.

Metal equipment, such as bed frames or curtain rails.—This should be cleaned daily with a damp duster, and washed with soap and water when necessary. A damp duster is used as it collects rather than scatters the dust. Ward cleaning is not normally carried out by the nursing staff, but they are responsible for seeing that it is done in the correct way.

Other hardware, e.g. washing bowls, is washed after use, scouring powder being used where necessary.

Wooden articles—lockers and bed tables.—These are damp

dusted daily and should be polished once or twice a week. Formica tops are wiped over with a damp cloth.

THE PATIENT'S DAY

Traditionally, the ward day starts early and to many patients is extremely tiring, owing to the incessant activity. In 1962, a Working Party report[1] emphasised the need for medical and nursing staffs to investigate conditions in their own hospitals; this has led, in many cases, to a rearrangement of work in an attempt to put the needs of the patient before the needs of the hospital.

Each 24-hour period naturally includes such normal activities as eating, washing and sleeping; in hospital, many investigations and treatments are added, together with the basic nursing care necessary for those confined to bed. This means that the patient's day is interrupted by a series of visits by various members of the hospital team; it is especially important to preserve the patient's rest hour in the middle of the day, to see that his mealtimes are uninterrupted and to ensure that his sleep is disturbed as little as possible.

The care of the seriously ill patient should be planned by all those who are concerned, e.g. doctor, nurse and physiotherapist, so that he is disturbed as infrequently as possible.

For convalescent patients and those needing little detailed nursing care, it is possible to reduce the number of routine procedures previously thought necessary; for example, many patients need only have their temperature, pulse and respiration rates taken and recorded once a day, and their beds can be made while they are up during the afternoon.

Many hospitals still have fixed visiting times, commonly in the early evening during the week, and in the afternoon at weekends. This has certain disadvantages in that it may be inconvenient for patients' relatives and friends and can be tiring for the patient in that the visitor usually feels that he must stay till the end of visiting time, even though the conversation may be exhausted and the patient wish to sleep. To overcome these difficulties, the Secretary of State has suggested more flexible visting hours and this is being carried out by several hospitals.

[1] H.M.S.O., *The Pattern of the In-Patients Day.*

Chapter IV

GENERAL CARE OF THE SICK

1. CARE AND COMFORT

Bedmaking

In an average ward some $\frac{2}{3}$ of the patients get up for part of the day; the beds of these patients are normally made once in 24 hours, during the time that they are unoccupied. As the remaining patients do not get up, their beds will be made more frequently.

Methods of bedmaking vary greatly from hospital to hospital, but the principles on which they are all based are the same. Provided these principles are adhered to, the details of the method used are unimportant.

The aim of bedmaking is to make the patient comfortable and to leave him refreshed and relaxed in a suitable position. To achieve this, the top bedclothes are removed, avoiding undue exposure of the patient, and a blanket or flannelette sheet is left to keep him warm while the bottom of the bed is being made. It is easier to proceed if the backrest—if used—and most of the pillows are removed, leaving the patient able to move, or be moved, from one side to the other; if for any reason he is uncomfortable or distressed when lying down, he should be left in the sitting position and moved as necessary. The bottom of the bed is remade in such a way that the bedclothes are taut and free from crumbs, hair clips and other debris; clean linen is used where necessary. The backrest and pillows are replaced, making sure that the patient is well supported, particularly in the hollows of the back and neck; the top pillow should be the softest available. The remaining bedclothes are replaced, care being taken to see that the patient's movements will not be restricted in any way. To avoid undue pressure on the feet he can be asked to cross his ankles while the top bedclothes are being replaced. If he is being nursed in a sitting position, the nurse must be careful that the bedclothes cover his chest. Before leaving the bedside, she must check that he is comfortable and that his locker and personal belongings are within easy reach.

Bedmaking provides an ideal opportunity to talk to the patient, since it usually involves two nurses being at the bedside for several minutes. Many patients welcome this contact and may, in the course of conversation, indicate some problem or symptom which has been worrying them. Should this be relevant to the patient's treatment or condition, it must be reported to the ward sister; otherwise it must be treated as a confidence.

Many patients are heavy and unable to move themselves; in this case the nurse must know how to lift and move them, without discomfort to the patient or injury to herself. During bedmaking, a helpless patient should be supported at all times, whether being moved from side to side or lifted. It is important to observe the position of the limbs, making sure they are in a natural position and not subject to unnecessary pressure.

There are two standard methods of lifting; in the first and older method, two nurses face each other across the bed; they grasp each other's hands or wrists at the bottom of the patient's back and under his thighs and lift together.

The other method is known as the Australian, or shoulder lift (see pictures—Fig. 6). This method has been shown to have many advantages, but cannot be used for patients with injuries, or who have had surgery of the chest, shoulder or upper arm.

In both methods of lifting the nurse's posture is important, in order that the strain is taken by the large muscles of the back and thighs, and not the small muscles of the shoulders or arms. The correct stance is with the feet apart, the knees and hips bent and the back straight.

The spread of infection from one patient to another is one of the problems in hospital wards. It has been shown that many bacteria may be transferred during bedmaking, as these are present in the dust and on the blankets themselves. To prevent dissemination care is necessary in the handling of all bed linen, and vigorous shaking is to be avoided. No articles should be put on the floor, or on other patients' beds. Soiled linen is placed in the appropriate container and should be sent to the laundry without further handling.

Bedmaking may be tiring, but the nurse can lessen fatigue by having all linen and equipment available before starting; most methods of bedmaking are designed to cut out unnecessary

35

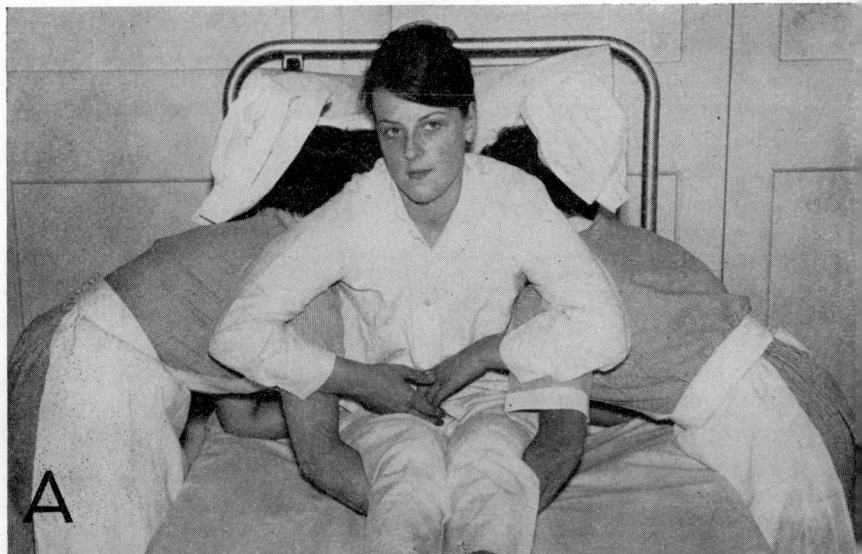

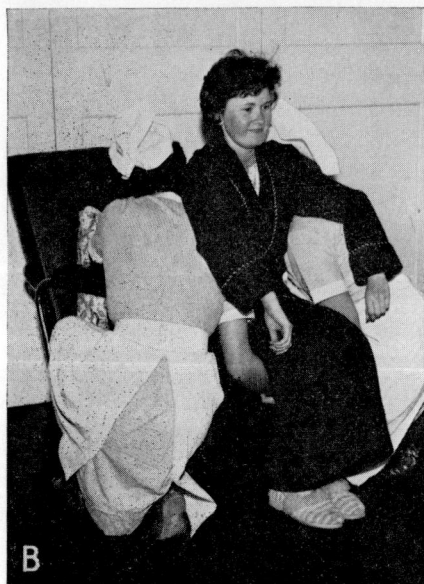

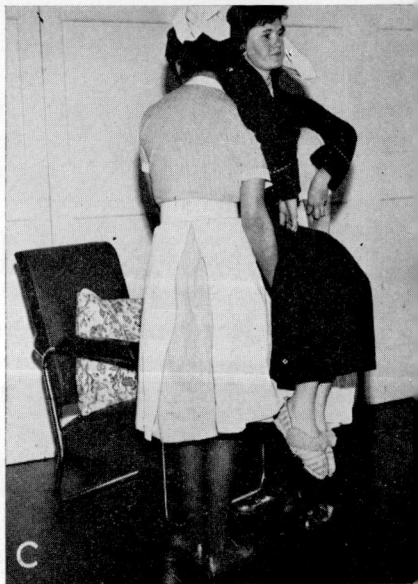

Fig. 6.—Lifting and Moving Patients.
A. In Bed.   B and C. From a Chair.

movement and, as mentioned, lifting patients properly will avoid strain.

In the past much emphasis has been placed on the tidiness of the beds, especially just before a doctor's round. A very untidy bed is often uncomfortable and this is a valid reason for tidying it; however, the appearance of the ward should not take precedence over the patient's comfort.

The use of accessories

Various aids to patient comfort include:

(a) **Backrests.**—These are usually part of the bed frame, and with pillows help to support the patient in a sitting position. For beds without a backrest, a portable one is used. Some more expensive, modern beds do not have a fixed back rest as such, but the top of the bed can be raised, so supporting the patient's head and shoulders.

(b) **Bed cradles.**—These are made of metal and are placed in the bed to take the weight of the bedclothes from a painful or injured part, or to allow the circulation of air. Since this raises the bed-clothes, it is often desirable

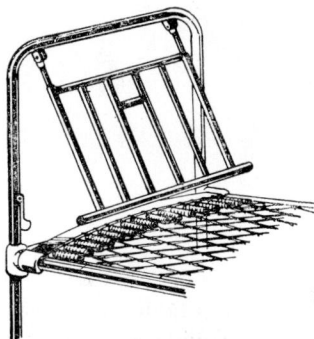

Fig. 7.—Fixed backrest (*Hoskins & Sewell Ltd.*).

to put a thin blanket or flannelette sheet next to the patient to keep him warm. During bedmaking, care must be taken when removing or replacing the cradle to avoid hurting the patient.

(c) **Air and water pillows and rings.**—These are rubber rings or pillows which are filled with air or water, placed in a cotton cover, and used for patients to sit or lie on. When placing them under a patient, the metal nozzle should be at the side, so that it does not cause discomfort. The amount of air or water used is important, too little or too much being useless and uncomfortable; although this will vary with the weight of the patient, the nurse

37

should experiment for herself in the practical classroom.

Sorbo-rubber rings are now more common and with the increasing number of interior sprung or similar mattresses, air and water pillows are less frequently used.

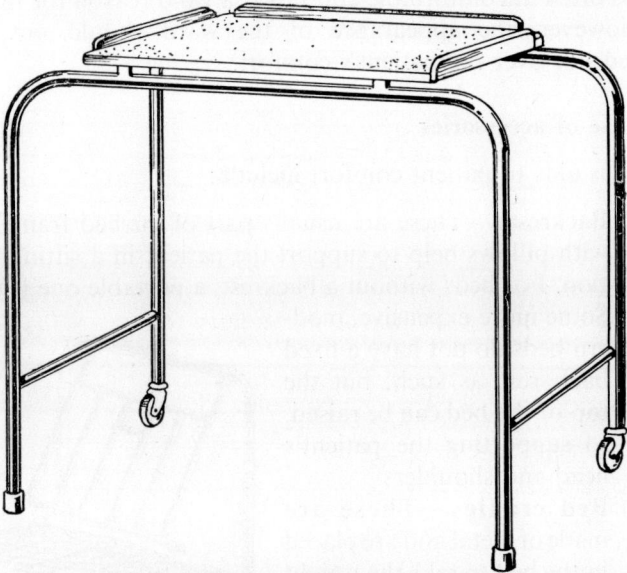

FIG. 8.—Bed Table (*Hoskins & Sewell Ltd.*).

(d) **Bed tables** are movable tables which fit over the bed and provide a surface for occupational therapy, meal trays or patients' belongings. Some modern lockers obviate the need for these, having a hinged flap, which when brought up extends over the bed. It is a great advantage if the height of the bed table can be adjusted.

(e) **Bed elevators.**—It is convenient to mention these here, although they are used more in treatment than as an aid to comfort. Wooden blocks, or a metal elevator, raise the foot or head of the bed by 6 inches to 2 feet as desired. Some modern beds have a lever and winding device, which when used raises or lowers the height of the bed or, if adjusted, either end of the bed.

(f) **Bed sides.**—It is necessary at times to attach padded boards or similar equipment to the sides of the bed to prevent a restless patient from falling out.

38

Positions used in nursing

The following positions may be used for the comfort and in the treatment of patients, examples being given in each case.

(a) **Recumbent (supine).**—The patient lies flat on his back— 1 pillow may be allowed.

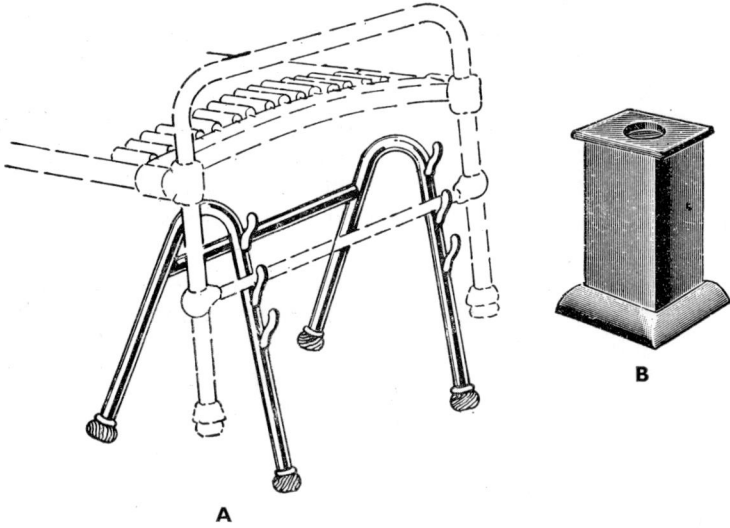

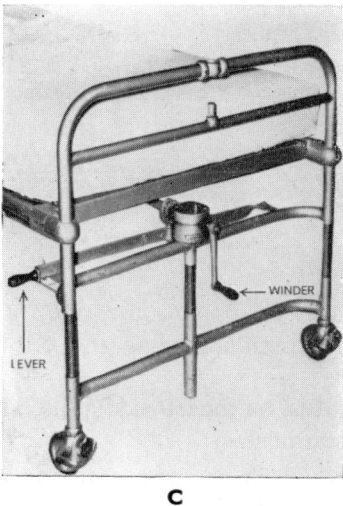

FIG. 9.—A. Portable Bed Elevator (*Hoskins & Sewell Ltd.*).
B. Block (*Chas. F. Thackray Ltd.*).
C. Fixed Bed Elevator (*J.Nesbit-Evans*)

Uses.—During examination by the doctor and for nursing procedures, such as the removal of stitches from an abdominal wound.

(*b*) **Semi-recumbent.**—A common position in which the patient is made comfortable with 2 or 3 pillows.

(*c*) **Sitting.**—This is self-explanatory.

Uses.—Following most abdominal operations, and for any patient having respiratory difficulty. This position is maintained by the use of several pillows and a backrest. A foot support may be necessary.

(*d*) **Prone.**—The patient lies face downwards; the position may be made more comfortable by the use of soft pillows under the chest, hips and ankles. Although this may look uncomfortable, it is surprising how quickly a patient will adapt to it.

Uses.—In severe burns or other injuries of the back.

(*e*) **Semi-prone.**—This position is best understood by referring to the picture below.

Uses.—In the immediate post-operative period (especially after tonsillectomy).

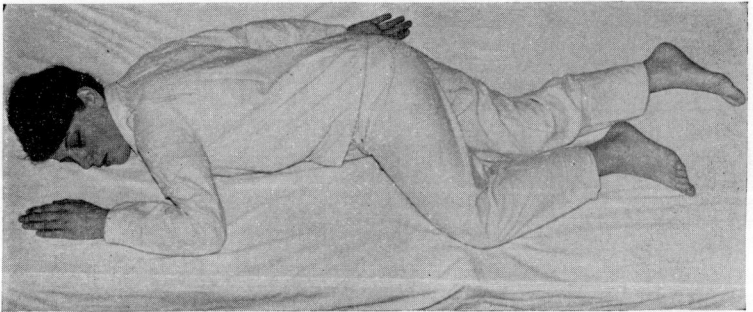

FIG. 10.—The Semi-prone Position.

(*f*) **Lateral.**—The word means "relating to the side" and this position is extremely common, being the one in which most people sleep.

Uses.—The left lateral (that is, on the left side) is used for rectal examination and treatment.

In all these positions it must be emphasised that the placing

40

of the patient's limbs is of great importance, and that during treatment or examination he should be exposed as little as possible.

Relief of pain; rest and sleep

It is not proposed to discuss the many drugs available for the relief of pain, but to indicate simple nursing measures which, by making the patient more comfortable can lessen pain or discomfort and help him to rest or sleep.

It is often found that a change of position will ease tension, as in many cases the patient is either afraid or unable to move himself without the nurse's assistance, particularly after surgery.

Other factors which may well cause discomfort are a full bladder or rectum; urinals or bedpans should be offered and a report made to the ward sister if no relief is obtained.

Many patients with high temperatures perspire profusely, and in this case the nurse may be asked to sponge the patient with cool water and to change his pyjamas and bed linen where necessary.

The patient may simply be too hot or too cold—in which case blankets should be removed as desired or additional warmth provided. Headaches are common if the atmosphere is stuffy; the nurse can do much to relieve this by adjusting the ventilation and so the temperature of the ward.

During the night, problems and worries become magnified out of all proportion and may well be the cause of insomnia. This is particularly true of patients who are shortly to have an operation, or who have been admitted as emergencies during the previous day. The nurse can often help by explanations, sympathy and understanding, and for those patients who are frightened a calm and confident manner is in itself reassuring.

A hot drink is often very acceptable to a sleepless patient.

A hospital ward appears strange to the new patient for the first few nights following admission. The nurse must remember that he is probably accustomed to the darkness and privacy of his own bedroom, and that it is an unusual experience for him to share his "bedroom" with 20 to 30 other people, some of whom may snore or be sick. However quietly the nurses move around the ward, a certain amount of noise is inevitable, especially if patients are admitted and/or go to the operating theatre. It is scarcely surprising that for many these first nights in hospital bring only fitful sleep.

Uses of heat and cold

The heat-regulating centre of the body is situated in the brain and in health the temperature varies very little even in hot or cold weather.

Heat is lost partly through the skin, due to the evaporation of sweat and to alterations in the amount of blood circulating in the superficial vessels. If these vessels dilate, more blood is brought near to the surface, the skin is flushed and feels warm and heat is lost to the atmosphere; if the vessels constrict—as in cold weather—less blood can flow through them, the skin looks pale and feels cold, and heat is retained. Heat is also lost in the urine and faeces and in expired air.

Heat is produced in the body during the breakdown of food and by the activity of glands, particularly the liver. Clothing is used as protection against extremes of temperature: in summer, light colours and thin materials help to keep the body cool; in winter darker colours and thicker materials are more suitable.

In hospital heat and cold are used to make the patient more comfortable, to relieve pain and to produce an alteration in body temperature if this is desired in treatment—an example of this is hypothermia, where the patient's temperature is lowered by the use of ice and fans.

Local applications of heat and cold act simply by dilating or constricting the surface blood vessels, so producing the changes described earlier.

These include:

Heat. 1. *Hot-water bottles.*—These are common aids to comfort in the home, but their use in hospital has declined, partly due to research into the physiology of shock and partly because of misuse. Hospital rules vary, but it is always wise to ask the sister-in-charge before giving a hot-water bottle to a patient. If one is allowed, it is advisable to place it on a flat surface and to fill it with hot (not boiling) water using a funnel—this lessens the risk of injury to the nurse; it should be tested for leakage, dried, put in a cover and placed between two of the blankets rather than next to the patient. Empty hot-water bottles are best stored slightly inflated, and should be hung from a hook rather than laid flat.

The following patients should not be given hot-water bottles —those with loss of sensation, the mentally confused, the unconscious or the paralysed, and small children.

Occasionally hot-water bottles are given to relieve pain.

2. *Electric pads and blankets.*—These may be used to warm a bed before a patient is admitted or returns from the operating theatre; this routine varies greatly and the wishes of the particular physician or surgeon must be observed. If they are used, they should always be removed before the patient is placed in bed.

When not in use, they are stored flat and in a dry place; the flex and plug must be checked at intervals by the electrician; where specific instructions from the makers are on the apparatus these should be observed.

3. *Poultices.*—Poultices have been used as a method of applying heat for hundreds of years; they are also used to localise infection—as in boils. Many types (bread, bran) have fallen into disrepute; the most common substance in current use is kaolin (Antiphlogistine)—a mixture of clay, aromatic oils and salicylates.

To make a poultice, the mixture is heated by standing the tin in hot water; it is then spread on a piece of old linen and may be covered with a thin layer of gauze.

Before applying it to the patient's skin, the nurse should see that it is not too hot by testing it on the skin of her own forearm; it is then applied, covered with a layer of cotton wool and bandaged lightly in position; it should be renewed when necessary. Kaolin is used as it retains heat well, and so is effective for a number of hours.

Cold. 1. *Cold compress.*—These are used to relieve pain due to congestion of a part, as in headache or a sprain. Pieces of old linen are wrung out in iced water and applied to the skin. They will need to be renewed frequently. Evaporating substances such as eau-de-Cologne, or a mixture of equal parts of methylated spirit and water, have the same effect.

2. *Ice poultice.*—This can be used to lessen bleeding—particularly from the nose. Very small pieces of ice are placed between 2 thin layers of cotton wool; this is then covered with thin polythene or other waterproof material, the edges being sealed, e.g. with Sellotape.

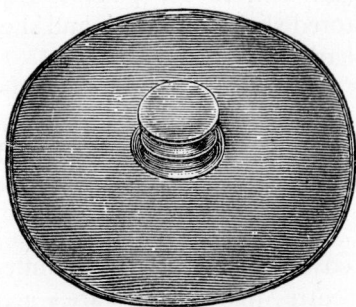

FIG. 11.—Ice Bag (*Allen & Hanburys*).

3. *Ice bags.*—Used mainly to lower the body temperature. Ice is broken into small pieces and put in the bag; the stopper is replaced firmly, and the bag put in a cover. It is usually suspended from a cradle, over the affected part, or occasionally may be placed on the skin, the site being changed frequently.

2. PERSONAL NEEDS

Under normal circumstances the skin, mouth and hair are cared for by a daily routine which, through the years, becomes a habit requiring little conscious thought.

It has already been emphasised that an important function of the skin is to produce sweat and so help to regulate body temperature; it is not always realised that at least 600 mls. of fluid is lost in perspiration every 24 hours, this amount being increased in hot weather and during exercise. Although there are sweat glands in all parts of the skin, they are more numerous in certain areas, e.g. the axillae, groins and soles of the feet. Frequent washing is not only refreshing but necessary to prevent body odour due to the decomposition of sweat, and to remove dirt and flakes of skin which are continually being shed.

In this country the traditional way of washing the whole body is to have a bath; while to us this is natural, people in other countries regard it as a rather unhygienic practice and prefer to take showers, which use less hot water and wash the dirt away from the skin.

Bathing in the bathroom and in bed

Patients allowed up for washing and toilet purposes will probably bath in the bathroom. It is not usual for the bathroom door to have a lock, so a screen inside, or an "Engaged" notice, is essential.

The nurse's responsibilities vary with the patient's capabilities, and the ward sister will indicate the amount of supervision needed. For those requiring assistance the nurse should prepare the room, the bath and the patient. Windows are closed, a chair and bath mat placed in position and the water run until the bath is one-third to half full; the temperature of the water is checked to make sure that it is neither too hot nor too cold, the nurse remembering that the skin of the hand is not a reliable guide. Where bath thermometers are used these should read 41° to 43° C. (105° to 110° F.); this thermometer has no constriction between the bulb and the shaft and must be read while the bulb is still well below the surface of the water.

The patient is assisted from his bed to the bathroom, all toilet requisites being collected from his locker. Pyjamas are placed on the radiator to warm, and if necessary the patient is helped into the bath. Where a male patient needs assistance or supervision it is customary for a male nurse or orderly to accompany him; in the case of female patients the nurse will stay. Although some patients can be left alone, it must be remembered that they may feel faint or need help, and it is reassuring for them to know that the nurse is within call.

If the patient is to return directly to bed, this is an opportunity for re-making it, using clean linen. When he has finished his bath and is warm and comfortable in a chair or in bed, the nurse returns to the bathroom, opens the windows, cleans the bath and sees that all the patient's personal belongings are put back in his locker.

A small number of patients, including the acutely ill, will be bathed in bed and this is carried out, ideally, every day. As with bedmaking, it provides an opportunity to increase the patient's comfort and to talk to him.

Many patients welcome the idea of a bath when it is explained to them, and the nurse then prepares the equipment and the bed. As far as equipment is concerned, the articles necessary are the normal toilet requisites; they will be found in the patient's locker.

It is usual and convenient to place these on a trolley, as the locker and bed table may be covered with the patient's personal belongings. A well filled bowl of hot water is necessary, the nurse remembering that few things are more uncomfortable than a tepid wash. Curtains are drawn round the bed and draughts excluded; the patient should be offered a bedpan or urinal.

The top bedclothes are removed and the patient covered with a blanket or flannelette sheet. In many hospitals a second flannelette sheet is rolled under the patient, because it feels warmer and absorbs water. His pyjamas (or nightgown) are removed and he is washed. Provided certain points are borne in mind, this is a straightforward procedure:

(a) Many people—especially women—do not like soap on their face; ask the patient.

(b) While the patient is being bathed he should be exposed as little as possible to avoid chilling; and also some people are embarrassed at the idea of being washed by another person.

(c) Each part of the body is washed in turn, using a well-soaped flannel; the area is then rinsed and dried thoroughly. When washing the hands and feet it is refreshing for the patient to put them in the bowl of water, this being placed on the bed. The nails are attended to where necessary.

(d) Special care must be taken where two skin surfaces meet, e.g. the axillae, and when washing the umbilicus. If the patient is able, he may prefer to dry himself, and he will almost certainly prefer to wash and dry the genital area himself.

(e) The water is changed when it becomes too soapy or dirty.

Although the patient will have to be turned to have his back washed, the nurse should remember that unnecessary movement will be tiring for him.

When the bath is finished, the pyjamas are put on again, the flannelette sheets removed and the bed remade with clean linen. The patient's mouth and hair are then attended to. Personal belongings are returned to the locker which is left within his reach. The curtains are drawn back and the remaining equipment is cleared away.

During her training the nurse will meet patients who for various reasons have not been able to maintain a high standard of personal hygiene; in the majority of cases this is not their fault. For example, elderly people with physical disabilities may appear neglected because they are unable to care for themselves as they would wish. Other patients come into hospital as the result of accident or sudden illness and have had no opportunity to prepare for admission; they are often distressed at this and need reassurance.

Special care of the skin

Everyone is familiar with the appearance of the skin if it is subjected to undue pressure; we have all at some time noticed the reddening and soreness of the elbows after resting on them while reading in bed, or at a table. This problem is magnified for those confined to bed, since it affects many areas not normally subject to long periods of pressure. These areas are called, appropriately, pressure areas, and include the elbows, shoulder blades, the spine in thin people, the buttocks, hips, knees, heels and ankles; it will be realised that these are all parts of the body where bony prominences are near the skin. Obviously the position of the patient determines which part is affected at any time.

If pressure to any area is not relieved at regular intervals, the circulation is interfered with and the nutrition of the cells is affected; the result of this process is reddening of the skin and subsequent tissue breakdown; this is then called a pressure sore. The process is hastened if the tissues are already undernourished due to the patient's illness. Other factors contributing to tissue breakdown are:

1. Moisture.
2. Friction, e.g. from crumbs, creases in the bottom bedclothes, or skin surfaces rubbing together.
3. Damage to the skin, e.g. by the careless removing of bedpans.

Certain patients may develop sore areas more quickly than

others. These include the thin—because there is little subcutaneous tissue between the bones and the skin; the fat—because of the extra weight; the paralysed and the unconscious—because they are unable to move themselves; and patients who have no control over their bladder (incontinent patients) —because the skin is continually wet.

If the predisposing factors in pressure-sore formation are understood, methods of prevention will be obvious. Before summarising these, it cannot be emphasised too strongly that it is far easier to prevent a pressure sore developing than it is to heal one once it has formed. A few hours' neglect can cause a lesion which will take weeks or even months to cure, adding not only to the patient's discomfort, but to the length of his stay in hospital.

Prevention of pressure sores

1. Movement: if the patient is unable to move himself, his position must be changed at least every 2 hours; in special cases it may be necessary more frequently than this. It is a good thing for the nurse to develop the habit of moving the patient to a new position whenever she attends to his needs.
2. Cleanliness and dryness; cleanliness of the skin has already been discussed—this is particularly important in the incontinent, whose care is given later in this chapter.
3. Care in bedmaking, and the use of bed accessories to relieve pressure.
4. Diet. If the patient is not eating a normal diet, the missing factors must be given in some form, e.g. high-protein milk and/or vitamin tablets.

The development of special mattresses has helped the nurse in caring for those patients in whom pressure sores are likely to develop. The "ripple" bed is an example; here the mattress is divided into sections and air is pumped continuously from one section to another; this causes a rippling movement on the surface of the mattress and constantly changes the areas subject to pressure.

Another aid is the use of a special bed-pad on which the patient lies or sits; originally, sheep-skins were used for this purpose, but now pads made from acrilan fibre are available.

These have a thick pile, and while they are very comfortable and distribute pressure evenly, they allow free circulation of air, are easily washed and sterilised, and will not support bacterial growth. Even when the patient is incontinent they do not become stained, and do not lose their soft texture with use. The pad is simply placed under the patient in direct contact with the skin.

In some hospitals the pressure areas are "treated" at regular intervals. This procedure consists of washing the skin, massaging the area to promote the circulation and sometimes applying

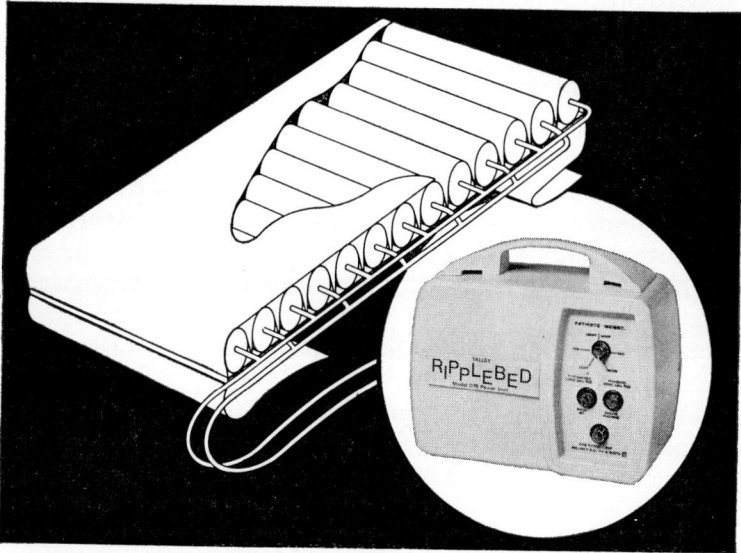

FIG. 12.—"Ripple" Bed (*Talley Surgical Instruments Ltd.*).

various lotions to harden the skin. It must be realised that in effect this treatment is simply a way of carrying out the measures described above, i.e.:

1. Movement—since the patient is moved to wash the area and the position changed.
2. Cleanliness and dryness.
3. Bedmaking—as during the procedure the bottom bedclothes are straightened.

Early recognition of the effects of pressure is important; the patient may complain of soreness or a tingling sensation, or the nurse may notice redness—this is a danger sign and should be reported. Provided the pressure is relieved, no further deterioration will occur; if it continues, the area will become blue and the skin will break.

One of the functions of the intact skin is to act as a barrier, and if it is broken bacteria can enter the tissues and cause infection. Because of this, it is essential to treat pressure sores, if they occur, as open wounds and to cover them with sterile dressings. A variety of lotions may be used, examples being aserbine, because of its cleansing action, and aqueous hibitane. It is also important to see that the patient does not lie on the affected area, as pressure lessens the blood flow to the part and further delays healing.

Care of the incontinent patient

Once control of the bladder has developed—at approximately 18 months of age—the passing of urine (micturition) is a voluntary act. In seriously ill or old people this control may be lost, urine being passed at intervals into the bed. Apart from the distress and discomfort to the patient, which may be considerable, this affects the skin as described earlier. Whenever it becomes wet it is most important to change the bed linen; at the same time the surrounding skin is carefully washed and dried, as urine acts as an irritant. To replace the natural oils lost from the skin as the result of incontinence, various creams, ointments or oils can be applied; these include zinc and castor oil cream, olive oil and "barrier" or silicone creams, which also serve as a waterproof covering. The makers of barrier creams usually give instructions as to their application and use—some being used only once in 24 hours.

Disposable incontinence pads may be placed under the patient; these consist of layers of absorbent material with a non-absorbent backing, and are used to lessen the amount of wet linen. Obviously they are changed when wet.

Bedpans should be offered at frequent intervals as the patient is unaware of the need to pass urine. Faecal incontinence may also be present and is discussed on page 139.

Care of the mouth

The mouth is a cavity lined by mucous membrane and is the beginning of the alimentary (digestive) tract. It is kept moist by saliva which is a watery fluid produced by glands, whose ducts open into the floor and sides of the cavity; the flow of saliva is increased by the sight, smell and taste of food, and by the action of chewing. The tongue is a muscular structure, playing an important part in speech and having special cells on its upper surface—the taste buds. The teeth are necessary for the breaking up of food and need care if they are to remain healthy.

In babies, the mouth needs little attention and is best left alone. Once teeth appear, regular brushing should be encouraged and visits to the dentist at 6-monthly intervals are advisable from an early age—$2\frac{1}{2}$ to 3 years. It is not always possible to brush the teeth after every meal, but it is important to do this before going to bed, and not to eat sweets afterwards. The amount of dental decay in schoolchildren is extremely high at present, and is probably due to lack of care and to an increase in the amount of sweets eaten. The type of toothpaste used is relatively unimportant, but a good toothbrush which is neither too hard nor too soft is an essential. The permanent teeth begin to erupt at about the age of 6, and the set is complete in the early 'teens. With care they will last for many years, and are usually much more satisfactory than the third set available under the National Health Service. Dentures need cleaning as much as natural teeth, but are removed for this purpose. Many proprietary pastes and powders are available, and some people leave their false teeth soaking in a cleansing solution overnight; the mouth is rinsed with water or a mouthwash when necessary.

In illness it is not always as easy to keep the mouth clean; the normal flow of saliva may be interfered with, and the mouth becomes dry. This is more likely in:

1. Those patients who have a high temperature.
2. Those who, for any reason, are unable to eat or drink as much as usual, or who have simply lost their appetites.
3. Patients who are vomiting excessively.
4. Unconscious patients, particularly those who breathe through their mouths, so causing drying of the mucous membrane.
5. Certain infections or conditions of the mouth itself.

Methods of cleaning the mouth and teeth.—The majority of patients will clean their teeth in the normal way in the morning and evening, the nurse providing the equipment for those confined to bed; it may be easier to clean dentures under a running tap.

For those in whom special care is needed, the nurse will be asked to give mouthwashes more frequently. Water is a perfectly adequate fluid for this purpose, but a pleasant colour and taste appeals to many patients; most hospitals have their own stock mouthwash, a common solution being glycerine and thymol (glycothymoline). The following help to keep the mouth moist and in some cases promote the flow of saliva:

Normal saline (1 teaspoonful of salt 600 mls. of water).
Fruit juices—particularly lemon or lime.
Soda water.

Even if a patient is not allowed solid food, he can be given slices of fruit to chew (orange, pineapple or lemon) which will help to keep his mouth fresh.

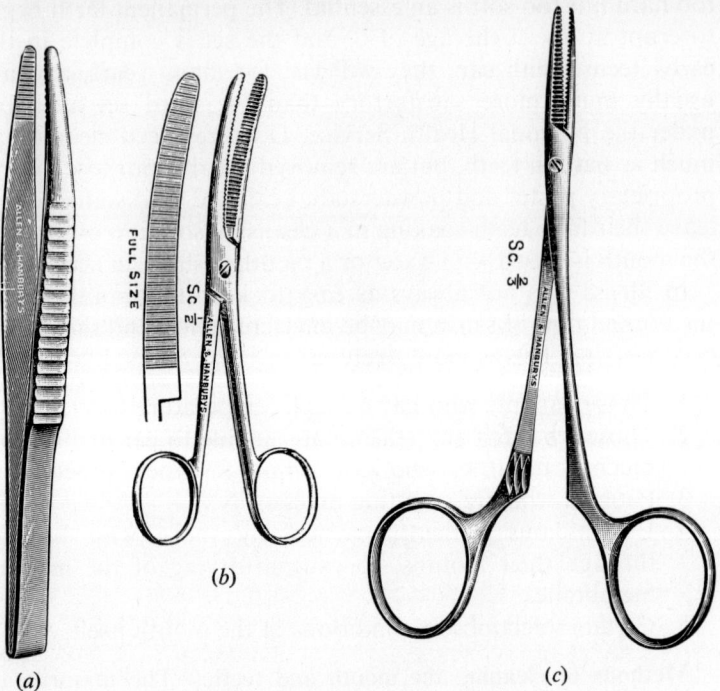

FIG. 13.—Forceps. (a) Dissecting, (b) Dressing, (c) Artery.

For a small proportion of patients it is necessary to use another method. This is sometimes referred to as special care, or swab cleansing.

The nurse explains what she is going to do, and draws the curtains or screens round the bed; the patient's gown and bedclothes are protected with a small towel. The nurse cleans the mouth, using swabs held securely in artery or dressing forceps.

The swab is dipped into a suitable lotion such as sodium bicarbonate, which has the property of dissolving dried mucus, and the inside of the mouth is swabbed; the swab is changed frequently, being removed from the holding forceps by means of dissecting forceps.

Care must be taken to avoid injury to the mucous membrane, and when cleaning the back of the tongue and soft palate which are particularly sensitive. Particles of food may be lodged between the teeth, and these can be removed with a dressed orange stick or wool carrier dipped in the cleansing lotion.

If the patient cannot use a mouthwash, the procedure is repeated using water or glycothymoline solution as a rinse. If the lips are dry, they can be lubricated with some ointment such as white petroleum jelly. The patient is left in a comfortable position, and the equipment is cleared away. Used swabs and orange sticks and any other disposable items are placed in the dirty dressing bag or bin, to be burned later in the hospital incinerator. The forceps and remaining equipment are washed in hot soapy water, rinsed, and either boiled in the ward steriliser for 5 minutes to kill any bacteria from the patient's mouth, or returned to the Central Sterile Supply Department (C.S.S.D.). It may be necessary to repeat this procedure every 2 to 4 hours.

The complications of a neglected mouth are:
Dryness, soreness and cracking of the lips;
Furred tongue;
Unpleasant taste leading to loss of appetite (anorexia);
Halitosis;
Infection of the structures within the mouth or those communicating with it, e.g. the parotid glands and the middle ear.

Care of the hair

The condition of the hair depends partly on the care it receives, and partly on the general health of its owner; normal care includes regular brushing and combing, which will be continued while the patient is in hospital. Cutting and washing are also necessary at intervals.

In many hospitals a barber visits the male wards to shave ill patients and to attend to their hair if necessary; as a man's hair is kept short, washing does not present a problem. For women, a hairdressing service may be provided; where this is not available, the patient who is allowed up can have her hair washed in the bathroom, the nurse helping her in the same way as she would help a friend in the nurses' home; patients normally like to provide their own shampoo. Occasionally, it may be necessary to wash the hair of a patient confined to bed; the most suitable position for the patient is sitting up and leaning forward over a washing bowl placed on the bed table. If she cannot sit up, the bowl is placed on the springs of the bed, as illustrated below, the mattress being pulled down about 18 inches.

The equipment includes an ample supply of hot water, which must be taken to the bedside, and waterproof covers to protect the patient and the bed. A flannel should be provided to cover the patient's eyes, and the temperature of the water carefully checked so that it is not too hot when it is poured on to the

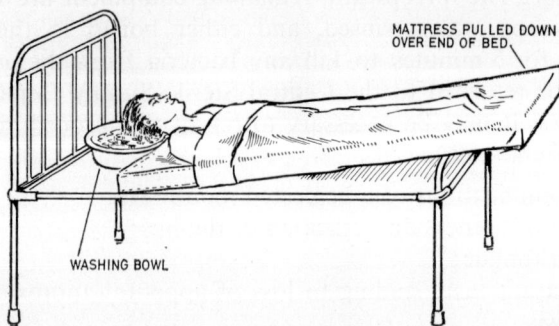

MATTRESS PULLED DOWN OVER END OF BED

WASHING BOWL

FIG. 14.—Washing Hair in Bed.

patient's head. On completion, the hair is dried, using towels and an electric hand drier, if available. It is set in a style which the patient likes.

In fact, in many hospitals, few patients are confined to bed long enough to make this necessary; however, many women are particular about their appearance and will be grateful for attention given. Well-dressed hair will do much to increase their morale, particularly before visiting hours.

Treatment of the infested head

Occasionally, due to neglect or poor social conditions, it is possible for the head to become infested with lice. These are tiny parasites which live on the human scalp, and obtain nourishment by biting. They lay eggs—called nits—which are attached to the hairs by a cement-like substance, and so grow out with them. The bites cause intense irritation which may lead to scratching and so to infection. The condition may be discovered—particularly in children—through irritability due to lack of sleep, and swollen glands at the back of the neck. It is contagious, being spread from one person to another by close contact, or sharing hats and combs.

This may be discovered by the nurse when she is admitting a new patient and, since it is more common in children, a closer scrutiny is necessary with this age group. Should she suspect infestation, it should be reported to the ward sister, who may ask her to fine tooth comb the patient's hair. Tact, understanding and privacy are necessary, as the patient may have no idea of the condition of her hair. During the process the comb is wiped on wool swabs which are then inspected; it is advisable to protect the patient's nightgown with a shoulder cape. If lice are found, the head will probably be treated with a solution of D.D.T., such as Suleo, or Dicophan; small quantities of the emulsion are applied, using swabs or a pipette, and massaged into the scalp; rubber gloves may be worn for this. The hair is left for 24 hours and then washed. If on further inspection nits are still present, vinegar may be added to the water to loosen the nits, which can then be removed by fine tooth combing. All equipment must either be disposed of, or washed, rinsed and sterilised; the combs may be placed in a suitable antiseptic solution—this varying according to local practice.

The use of bedpans and urinals

Urine is secreted by the kidneys and excreted from the

55

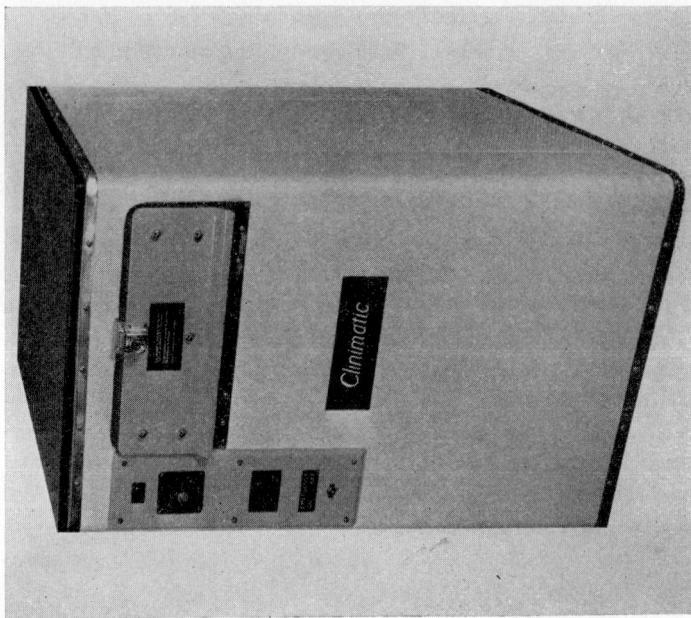

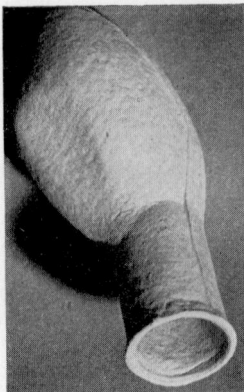

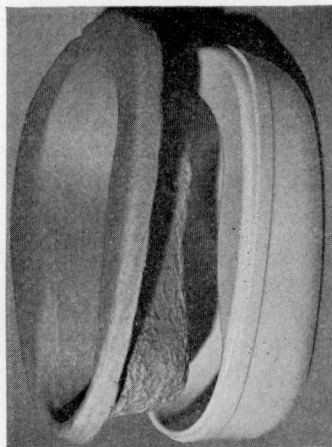

FIG. 5.—(a) Disposal machine for papier maché bedpans. (b) Disposable urinal. (c) Disposable bedpan and its fibreglass carrier (*Vernon & Co., Preston*).

56

bladder; it is a means by which the body loses fluid and certain waste products, e.g. urea and various salts. The average amount of urine produced in 24 hours is 1200–1800 mls., depending mainly on the amount of fluid drunk. Urine is passed 4 to 6 times each day, but this too is a variable, depending on nervousness, opportunity, the weather and other factors. The capacity of the bladder is about 600 mls. in the adult, although this can be greatly increased in certain conditions; the bladder responds to filling by stimulating nerve-endings which make us aware of our need to pass urine.

Faeces are semi-solids, consisting of water, cellulose (indigestible food), bacteria and cells shed from the lining of the alimentary tract. When the rectum is full, nerve-endings are stimulated, thus producing conscious sensation and the desire to defaecate; the bowels are usually opened once daily.

Perhaps the least acceptable part of the in-patient's routine is the bedpan. Wherever possible patients who cannot walk to the lavatory are assisted on to a commode, or taken to the toilet in a special chair; it is now realised that, although this means getting in and out of bed, it causes far less strain than using a bedpan.

For the few who must stay in bed, privacy and a warm, dry bedpan are needed, toilet paper being placed within reach; it is important to see that the patient is well supported and is as comfortable as possible; male patients who require a bedpan are given a urinal as well; afterwards a bowl of water is offered for the patient to wash his hands.

When a helpless patient is unable to attend to his own needs, the nurse must do this for him.

After handling bedpans or urinals, she must wash her hands.

Paper (disposable) bedpan covers are now replacing the old cotton squares; after removal, the bedpan should be covered and taken to the sluice where the contents are inspected, measured if necessary and disposed of, bedpan washers or sterilisers often being available. A modern development is the papier-mâché bedpan, but this requires special methods of disposal.

Although, traditionally, bedpans are offered to all patients at set times—usually after meals when they might be expected to use them—it must be realised that the bladder and bowels respond to nervous stimuli within the patient, and not only to ward routine; where set rounds are the pattern, the patient may worry about asking for a bedpan between times, and suffer considerable discomfort as a result.

Additional needs

In this chapter the patient's personal needs have been discussed; for those who are confined to bed there are dangers of which he is unaware, and from which the nurse must protect him. Briefly these arise from lack of movement, and apart from pressure sores include:

Foot drop;
Venous thrombosis;
Chest complications.

1. **Foot drop.**—The normal position of the foot is at right angles to the leg, this position being necessary for walking. If the muscles on the anterior surface of the foot and ankle become weak, the foot begins to "drop". This condition is hastened if the top bedclothes are pulled too tightly over the feet during bedmaking, so pushing them into an unnatural position. To prevent foot drop, the bedclothes should be tucked in loosely, and often some type of foot-rest is put in the bed to hold the feet upright. The following may be used for this purpose:

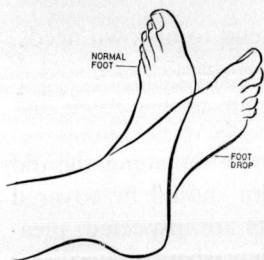

(*a*) Sandbags.

(*b*) A foot-board, kept in place by being slotted through a cradle.

(*c*) A small pillow, wrapped in a drawsheet, the ends of which are tucked under the mattress.

FIG. 16

2. **Venous thrombosis.**—The return of blood from the legs to the heart is facilitated by the continual movement of muscles which press on the veins in the calves. When a patient is sitting still in bed, the blood flow is slower owing to lack of movement, and pressure. Because of this a thrombus (or

clot) may form, and a piece break off and be carried in the blood stream (embolus), eventually blocking a major vessel, which is a serious and sometimes fatal condition. To prevent a clot forming, the legs must be moved at frequent intervals. If the patient is able, he must be encouraged to do this himself, and if not, the nurse or physiotherapist should carry out passive movements whenever the bed is made or attention given.

Should the patient complain of pain or tenderness in the calves, this must be reported immediately, as this, and an unexplained slight rise in temperature, may be the first signs of clot formation. Pillows or sandbags must never be placed under the knees or calves without being removed at regular intervals and the limbs exercised, as these will press on superficial vessels and increase the risk.

3. Chest complications.—A patient sitting or lying in bed tends to breathe less deeply than if he were up and about. This means that he is only using the upper part of the lungs, and in time the lower lobes may become "waterlogged" with secretions; this can lead to infections such as pneumonia. To prevent this, deep breathing and coughing should be encouraged, particularly if the movements are painful, as after high abdominal surgery. Alterations in position will also help.

It will be noted that in these conditions, as in pressure sores, prevention is better than cure. A short period of neglect can lead to a long period of pain and discomfort for the patient, and even failure to recover from the original illness. It is to prevent these complications that early ambulation following surgery has been introduced.

Chapter V

FOOD AND DRINK

Food is a topic which arouses interest in most people. As well as being necessary to maintain life, its consumption is a source of pleasure, the amount and type eaten depending, to a large extent, on locality, availability and income. In some cases, food eaten or avoided is not only a matter of personal preference, but of religious belief and custom; for example, the orthodox Jew must not eat pork, and to the Hindu the cow is a sacred animal; also many people are vegetarians.

Taste develops at an early age and the range of foods eaten and liked in later life will depend to a great extent on the foods given in childhood. Taste itself is confined to four sensations—these being appreciated by the taste buds in the tongue. They comprise sweet, salt, bitter and sour. All other flavours are in fact smells, interpreted by the brain, through experience—as specific foods. This fact will be obvious to anyone who has had a severe cold in the nose, when food appears tasteless.

Food eaten supplies the raw materials for growth and repair of tissues, and when burnt in the body produces heat and energy. The science of food and feeding is called nutrition, and in order to study food values more exactly a unit or measurement is required. This unit is the Calorie—this being the amount of heat needed to raise the temperature of 1 kg. of water 1° C.

The number of Calories required by each individual daily depends on size, age, sex and the amount of work to be done. To obtain the number needed, it is necessary to estimate the Basal Metabolic Rate—that is, the rate at which the body works when at rest and to add to this sufficient Calories to provide energy for all activities.

Examples of the number of Calories needed for certain activities are:

1. Sitting still   15 Cals./hour.
2. Standing   20 Cals./hour.
3. Sedentary occupation 25 to 30 Cals./hour.
4. Heavy manual work   320 Cals./hour.
5. Climbing   up to 960 Cals./hour.

Calories are obtained from:

Protein
Carbohydrate $\Big\}$ from foodstuffs
Fat
and Alcohol.

Other essential factors in food are:

Mineral salts
Vitamins
Water.

PROTEINS

These are complex body-building foods and are present in all living tissue. Chemically they consist of carbon, hydrogen, oxygen, nitrogen, sulphur and, in some cases, phosphorus; and are in fact the only source of the last three named. Proteins can be broken down into simpler units called amino-acids, of which some twenty-three are known. Of these nine are essential to life and cannot be obtained except from animal tissue; the others can be synthesised in the body.

Sources.—They may be obtained from animal or vegetable sources, and are found in the following foods:

1. Animal—lean meat, fish, cheese, eggs, milk.
2. Vegetable—beans, peas, nuts, whole-grain cereals and, therefore, flour.

Although the proportion of protein found in animal and vegetable foods is roughly the same, animal foods are of more value in that they contain the essential amino-acids; because of this, animal protein is sometimes called "first class".

Proteins provide 4·1 Calories per gramme weight (120 Cals. per ounce).

Protein cannot be stored in the body and so a regular intake is necessary. When it is digested and used there is a final waste product—urea—which is excreted in the urine. The amount of protein needed in the diet is approximately $\frac{1}{10}$ to $\frac{1}{8}$ of the total Calorie intake each day: it is recommended that half of this should be animal protein. These foods tend to be expensive.

61

CARBOHYDRATES

These are energy giving foods and form the largest part of the diet. They consist chemically of carbon, hydrogen and oxygen; are divided into sugars, starches and cellulose; and are all vegetable in origin.

Sugars are simple carbohydrates and can always be recognised because they taste sweet. Glucose, which is one of the simplest sugars, is the form in which carbohydrate is used in the body.

Starches are more complicated, being compounds of the simple sugars.

Other carbohydrates referred to as cellulose are the most complex type. They are plant cell wall products and are often called roughage. Although they have no food value, they form a useful part of the diet, providing bulk—so stimulating peristalsis.

Sources

Sugars: Fruits, honey, cane sugar.

Starches: Cereals, potatoes, root vegetables.

Cellulose: Raw vegetables and fruit.

In the body, carbohydrate is stored as animal starch—glyco-gen—in the liver and muscles. If too much is eaten, the excess is converted to fat and stored in the subcutaneous tissues.

Carbohydrates provide 4·1 Calories/gramme weight; 120 Calories/ounce.

Insulin (which is secreted by the pancreas) is needed for the utilisation of sugar in the body. There are no end products of metabolism except carbon dioxide and water. Carbohydrates tend to be cheap and are easily available. They make up approximately ⅗ of the total Calorie intake.

FATS

Fats provide heat and energy and consist chemically of carbon, hydrogen and oxygen. These form compounds known as glycerol and fatty acids; these acids are described as being saturated or unsaturated.

62

Sources of fats

Saturated: Milk, butter, fat meat.

Unsaturated: Olive oil, corn oil, nuts, oily fish (salmon, sardines, herrings).

The importance of this division lies in the fact that research has shown that too high a proportion of saturated fats may predispose to some types of heart disease, while unsaturated fats may lessen the risk.

Fats take longer to digest than other foods and also produce more Calories for the same weight:

1 gramme of fat yields 9·3 Calories.

1 ounce of fat yields 280 Calories.

When fats are metabolised (broken down and used) in the presence of sugar, the only waste products are water and carbon dioxide. If, however, sugar is not available, other products called ketones are formed which may be dangerous. This does not normally occur in the healthy person. Excess fat is stored in the subcutaneous tissues.

Fats form approximately $\frac{1}{3}$ of the total Calorie intake. Some fats contain other factors—the fat-soluble vitamins A, D, E, K.

MINERAL SALTS

These elements do not provide Calories but are essential for many body processes. They are needed in small amounts and, provided a satisfactory intake of proteins, fats and carbohydrates is maintained, no deficiency in salts is likely to occur.

Sodium and *chlorine* combine to form sodium chloride and as such are present in all body fluids. The amount found in the body is fairly constant and is closely linked with water balance: severe depletion, due for example to excess vomiting or diarrhoea, is a serious condition needing urgent treatment in the form of replacement therapy.

The amount of sodium chloride needed daily is 4 grammes, but most people eat far more than this, the average intake in a normal diet being 15 grammes. Excess is excreted in urine and sweat. Many foods, e.g. bacon, kippers, cheese, bread and cornflakes, contain salt, and more is added in cooking and at the table.

Potassium is found in most cells and is needed for the health of muscle and nerve tissue. The amount of potassium needed is about the same as sodium, and as it is found in most foods, no deficiency is likely to occur.

Calcium is necessary for the growth of bones and teeth, clotting of blood and contraction of muscles. Adults need approximately 1 gramme a day; children, adolescents and pregnant women requiring more. It is found in many foods, of which milk and cheese are the best sources. Its absorption and utilisation is complex and Vitamin D is necessary for the process.

Iron forms an essential part of red blood cells, combining with a protein to form haemoglobin: this is important as haemoglobin is the oxygen-carrying substance of the blood. Once iron is taken into the body it is retained and used again and again. A small amount is lost in daily wear and tear—and women lose some during menstruation. Because of this their intake needs to be higher than that of men. Obviously when bleeding occurs iron is lost in the red blood cells.

The daily requirement is small, being 12 to 15 mgms., and it is found in meat, particularly liver and kidney, tinned sardines and pilchards, cocoa and other foods. Milk contains practically no iron and since this is the staple food for babies, anaemia may occur if weaning is late. Iron deficiency is also found in adolescents, busy housewives and the elderly (amongst others) due to lack of attention to diet.

Phosphorus is needed with calcium for the formation of bones and teeth and many other processes. The ratio of calcium to phosphorus is 1:1·5, and a normal diet will provide a sufficient amount, since it is contained in milk, cheese, bread, eggs, potatoes and meat.

Many other minerals are needed in small amounts, but under normal circumstances deficiencies are unlikely to occur. These include iodine, magnesium, copper, zinc and fluorine.

ELECTROLYTES

During her training the nurse will often hear the term "electrolytes". This is used to describe certain compounds, e.g. sodium chloride, which, when dissolved in water, split up into their constituent elements, i.e. sodium and chlorine. This process is called ionisation, and because the elements taking part carry an electric charge, the term electrolytes is used. In fact, the main electrolytes are: sodium, potassium, chlorine and calcium, and it is when normal blood levels of these are altered that the patient is said to be in electrolyte imbalance. From a practical point of view this means replacement of fluid containing the deficient elements, usually intravenously.

VITAMINS

These are classified as being fat soluble or water soluble. The fat soluble are vitamins A, D, E and K, and the water soluble are the B group and vitamin C.

As with minerals, vitamins are needed in extremely small amounts, and are essential for certain body processes and for the health of the tissues. Many of the chemical reactions taking place in the body are influenced by enzymes and some of these cannot function alone, but require the presence of vitamins.

International Units are the agreed standard of measurement for many, as an indication of their value to the body.

Fat-soluble group

Vitamin A.—Many fruits and vegetables, e.g. carrots, spinach, watercress and apricots, contain a pigment, carotene, which gives them their colour; carotene, when taken into the body, can be converted into vitamin A. The animal sources of this vitamin are milk, butter, cheese, eggs and fish liver oils, and these are better sources, since man is not efficient at converting carotene.

It is essential for epithelial tissues, necessary for growth during childhood and is a constituent of the pigment which enables us to see in dim light.

Estimates of the amount of Vitamin A needed daily vary, but 4,000 I.U. is an average.

Vitamin D.—This is produced by the action of sunlight on the skin, and obtained from the intake of certain foods, e.g. dairy products and fish liver oils. Its absorption is closely linked with that of calcium and phosphorus, and it is necessary for growth and particularly the health of bones and teeth. The

65

daily intake needed from food is 200 I.U. in the adult, and more is necessary for children and pregnant women. However, it can be dangerous if babies are given too much vitamin D. A synthetic form is calciferol, which is obtainable as tablets.

Vitamin E.—Very little is known of this vitamin—it is found in milk and wheat germ, and as yet has little relevance in nutrition.

Vitamin K.—This vitamin is concerned with the normal clotting mechanism of blood: it is found in green vegetables, egg yolk and liver. It is also synthesised by bacteria in the gut and therefore in a healthy person deficiency is unlikely to occur.

Water-soluble group

The group of vitamins collectively called **B complex** comprise a number of substances often found in the same foods; some of the group are synthesised by bacteria in the gut. Only the more important will be mentioned by name.

Thiamine, nicotinic acid and riboflavine are necessary for growth, health of nerve tissue and epithelial tissue, and are found in wholemeal flour, yeast, eggs, green vegetables, milk and other foods.

The amounts needed daily vary and are measured in milli-grammes. These vitamins have now been added to many foods —i.e. "improved" flour and cornflakes.

Vitamin B12 is unlike the rest of the group. It plays an essential part in the formation of red blood cells and is present in animal foods—liver, meat, fish, eggs and milk.

Vitamin C.—Vitamin C, or ascorbic acid—is necessary for the health of small blood vessels and the healing of injured tissues. It is found in fresh fruit and vegetables, but as it is easily destroyed in cooking there may be a shortage in the food actually eaten.

The daily requirements are 20 to 40 mgm.—and excess is secreted by the kidneys.

WATER

Water is necessary for every body process although it provides no Calories. Chemically it is made up of hydrogen and oxygen, 1 molecule having the formula H_2O.

Approximately 70% of the body weight is water, and most of

this (50%) lies within the cells—the rest being extra-cellular and forming blood and the tissue fluids.

In health, the intake of fluid daily is equal to the fluid lost; if this balance is upset a patient either retains fluid and becomes oedematous (waterlogged), or loses excess amounts and becomes dehydrated.

Fluid intake

Fluid is gained by the body in 3 ways:

1. By drinking (water, tea, beer and other fluids).
2. In food, e.g. meat is 50% to 70% water; milk is 88% water.
3. Metabolic water: as referred to earlier, one of the products of carbohydrate and fat metabolism is water.

Fluid loss

Fluid is lost from the body in urine, sweat, faeces and expired air.

Approximate amounts:

Intake		Output	
Fluid drunk	1800 mls.	Urine	1800 mls.
Fluid in food	900 mls.	Sweat	600 mls.
Metabolic water	300 mls.	Expired air	450 mls.
		Faeces	150 mls.
3000 mls. = 3 litres		3000 mls. = 3 litres	

Although all the food factors have been considered separately, it is important to remember that any one food may contain many of them. In fact very few foods contain only one factor, exceptions being lard or cooking fat, which is 100% fat, and sugar which is 100% carbohydrate; no foods are 100% protein. An example of a food containing many factors is:

Bread	Protein	6%
	Fat	1·5%
	Carbohydrate	50%
	Minerals	Iron and Calcium
	Vitamins	B
	Water	42%

NORMAL NEEDS

It has already been mentioned that the number of Calories needed daily is the Basal Metabolic Rate in Calories, + Calories needed for activity. It is also important to bear in mind the individual's age, height, build and temperament, as these will influence their weight. For those over 40 years of age, the aim should be to keep the weight slightly below average, rather than above. Individuals vary greatly, but 20% above or below the average can be taken as being too fat or too thin. Violent changes in weight—particularly due to excessive slimming—can be harmful, unless carried out under medical supervision.

Examples of approximate Calorie intakes for different persons and ages are given below, and 2 menus, showing the amounts and types of food which will provide the Calories indicated.

Growing children: 35 to 50 Calories/pound of body weight/day according to age

Adolescents:	Boys:	3000 to 3500 Calories/day
	Girls:	2400 to 2600 Calories/day
Adults:	Sedentary occupation:	2000 to 2200 Calories/day
	Active occupation:	3000 to 4000 Calories/day
	Very active occupation:	3500 to 5000 Calories/day

Needs of the in-patient

Any establishment catering for a large number of people has to take into account the difficulties of satisfying individual tastes; in hospital this is made more difficult by the fact that many of the patients may have poor appetites, and some will have dietary restrictions because of their illness. In addition, there are problems with regard to transport of food from central kitchens to wards which are often widely scattered.

The head of the catering department, in most hospitals, is the catering officer who is responsible for the day to day running of the department, for the planning and preparation of food for the patients having normal diets, and often for the staff too. In some hospitals, special diets are planned and prepared in a separate department, under the supervision of dietitians. In hospitals where a dietitian is not employed, all food will be prepared in the main kitchen.

It is customary to discuss patients' diets under four headings: full, light, fluid and special.

Full diet.—This is suitable for those patients for whom no dietary restrictions are necessary, and is basically the same as one would eat at home.

Light diet.—This diet is suitable for those patients unable to eat a normal meal (full diet) and for whom no special diet has been ordered. It consists of easily digested foods such as chicken, boiled, steamed or grilled fish, minced lean meat, eggs in various forms, and mashed or sieved vegetables, followed by milk jellies or puddings, custards and ice cream. The term "bland" diet is used to describe non-irritating foods such as those mentioned above. It is sometimes difficult to provide colour and variety in light diets, but an effort must be made if the patient's appetite is to be stimulated.

Fluid diet.—This is, as its name implies, for patients unable to eat solid food. Its planning is usually the responsibility of the nursing staff, who prepare the necessary fluids in the ward kitchen, and supplement them with soups, which may be provided from the main kitchen. Jellies, ice cream and egg custards are often given, though not strictly fluids. When planning a fluid diet three considerations are important:

1. Fluid intake.
2. Calorie intake.
3. Food factors.

Milk is usually the basis of this diet, since it contains many food factors in their correct proportions. Minerals and vitamins can be given orally as ordered.

Special diets.—These are ordered for patients whose conditions necessitate some addition to, or restriction of, normal diet. The main ones are:

Low Calorie.
High or low protein.
Low fat.
Low sodium.
Low residue.
Diabetic.

69

Low Calorie.—The normal Calorie intake, as has been mentioned, is 2000 to 4000 per day. This may be reduced for patients who are overweight, the amount of carbohydrate and fat in the diet being restricted. If a patient is confined to bed, the reduction in Calories can be greater, as activity is less. Encouragement is often needed in the early stages of the diet, as it is extremely difficult for him to watch other patients enjoying a normal meal.

High protein.—The average daily intake of protein is 70 grammes. This may be increased for patients who need extra nourishment after prolonged illness and before or after major surgery. It must be remembered that a diet rich in all foodstuffs, especially protein, is essential to prevent sore pressure areas. Extra protein is also given to those suffering from certain types of kidney disorder when protein (albumin) is lost in the urine in large amounts.

Low protein.—It has already been mentioned that the end product of protein metabolism is urea which is excreted in the urine. If this mechanism is disturbed and urea retained, the amount of protein eaten must be restricted. The normal blood urea is 20 to 40 mgms. % (per 100 mls.).

Low fat.—Fat is restricted for patients with a tendency to certain types of heart disease in which fat is deposited along the walls of the arteries; associated with this is a raised blood cholesterol (normal 120 to 200 mgms. %). As mentioned before, the saturated fatty acids may be responsible for this and therefore it is advisable to restrict these. The total average daily intake of fat in health is 70 grammes, of which more than half may contain saturated fatty acids.

Low sodium.—Under normal conditions excess salt is lost from the body in urine and sweat. In circulatory and renal failure, salt and water may be retained in the body, resulting in oedema. The salt and water balance is so delicate that if the intake of salt is restricted, extra water is lost to restore the balance, so lessening the amount of fluid in the tissues. A low salt diet is one where salty foods are avoided, no extra salt is given, and in extreme cases salt is omitted from all cooking; in the latter case a salt substitute may be provided since the food will be quite tasteless.

Low residue.—The composition of faeces includes cellulose (roughage) which by its bulk stimulates peristalsis (movement of the gut) and so moves on the bowel contents. When the bowel wall is inflamed, roughage can be omitted from the diet to reduce undue stimulation. This is achieved by avoiding all foods containing cellulose; puréed fruits and vegetables are allowed because of their vitamin content.

Diabetic.—Patients suffering from diabetes mellitus have a deficiency of insulin resulting in defective carbohydrate and fat metabolism. For this reason it is necessary to modify the diet so that the amount of fat and carbohydrate are in the correct proportion, and are eaten at regular intervals. Daily injections of insulin may also be necessary.

Specimen diet sheets for a high-protein and a low-residue diet are provided; however, these are merely examples, as various combinations of special diets are often ordered.

PREPARATION FOR MEALS

Although meals in hospital follow the same pattern as those at home, i.e. breakfast, mid-morning drink, lunch, tea and supper, the time is usually rather earlier than that to which many patients are accustomed; this applies particularly to the evening meal which is often at 6 p.m. to 6.30 p.m.

Preparations for meals begin about half an hour before the food is served. Bedpans or urinals should be offered to those confined to bed, and washing bowls given afterwards, the nurse making sure that these patients are comfortable and in a suitable position for eating. It is more enjoyable to eat sitting at table, and it is usual to set one for those able to get up. Any medicines ordered to be taken before food should be given 20 to 30 minutes before the mealtime.

It is most important that the atmosphere should be as calm and relaxed as possible; in order to achieve this any dressings or treatments should be completed well in advance, and all activity in the ward reduced to a minimum. One of the reasons for nursing acutely ill patients in a side ward is to avoid the situation where their care disturbs other patients, and this is particularly important at mealtimes. The nurse is a vital part of the ward atmosphere and she too must appear calm and un-hurried; however busy her morning may have been, she should spare time to attend to her appearance and if possible and/or necessary put on a clean apron before handling food.

Other members of the ward team—i.e. auxiliaries or orderlies—will also have been getting ready in the kitchen; trays will have been laid with the appropriate cutlery and cruets, plates for hot food will be warming and serving spoons placed in readiness. It will be appreciated if someone checks that all patients who can, have water to drink with their meal.

SERVING MEALS

In most hospitals, food is delivered to the ward, by a kitchen porter, in heated trolleys, commonly called "hot locks", which can be plugged into the ward electricity supply.

The ward sister or her deputy usually serves the meal from this trolley, the patient's individual likes and dislikes being considered as far as possible. First helpings are usually quite small, as it is far better for the patient to feel he would like some more, than to be presented with a heaped plateful of food which may make him lose what little appetite he has. Gravy, vinegar, mint sauce and other condiments should be taken to the bedside for the patient to help himself if he wishes. It has been mentioned that plates are put to warm in preparation for the meal; obviously cold plates are used for cold food. It is preferable to take plates of food to the bedside on a tray, to avoid unnecessary handling. Second helpings are given as desired.

When all the patients are ready, dirty plates are collected; the ward sister is informed of any patient who has eaten little or nothing. No one should be made to feel that the nurse is in a hurry—even if she is!

Further courses are served in the same way.

Where possible, individual teapots are used, in preference to a communal supply; when these are not available, allowance must be made for variations in taste.

For those on special diets, it is essential to give the right diet to the right patient at the right time—and with these patients it may be even more important to note and report accurately on the amount of food eaten or refused—for instance, in a patient with diabetes mellitus. Fluid diets have already been mentioned; in these cases, patients may be ordered hourly or

2-hourly drinks, and these will be eagerly awaited and should not be delayed.

Any waste food is usually placed in a special bin—often being used for pig food; if this is so, tea leaves, orange peel and egg shells are disposed of separately.

FEEDING PATIENTS

In every ward there will probably be one or two patients unable to feed themselves—for instance, the very ill, the paralysed, patients with both eyes covered and those who are on complete rest. In these cases it is the nurse who will feed them.

The patient is made comfortable, and the pyjamas and top bedclothes are protected with a diet cloth. The nurse collects the food, making sure it is something the patient will eat, and seats herself comfortably at the bedside. Condiments are added as desired, and the patient offered small amounts of food on a spoon or fork. The meal should be unhurried, the patient being given drinks when he wishes, and the opportunity taken to talk to him. Most adults dislike being fed and the nurse's attitude will make a great deal of difference as to whether he enjoys the meal. When a patient is unable to see, he will appreciate being told in advance what he is going to eat.

HIGH-PROTEIN DIET
Approximately 90 grammes

On waking	Tea with milk from allowance (1,000 mls.).
Breakfast	Coffee with milk from allowance.
	Cereal with milk from allowance.
	or porridge
	Bacon and egg or scrambled egg.
	or smoked haddock.
	or cold ham.
	Bread or toast with butter and marmalade.
Mid-morning	Milk from allowance (flavour as desired).
	Biscuits—plain or sweet.
Lunch	Good helping of meat/fish/poultry.
	or omelette with cheese.
	Vegetables and potatoes.
	Milk pudding or egg custard/fruit and custard /sponge pudding (made with eggs).

Tea	Tea with milk.
	Sandwiches with egg or meat paste/ham/sardines/ cheese.
	Cake if desired.
Supper	Egg dishes/cheese pudding/cheese custard/fish, poultry or veal dishes.
	Vegetables.
	Egg custard, or milk jelly/fruit mousse/ice cream.
	Tea or coffee if desired.
Bedtime	Milk drink—flavoured as desired.
	Biscuits—plain or sweet.
Supplements	Fruit, chocolate, fruit juices.

LOW-RESIDUE DIET

On waking	Tea.
Breakfast	Tea or coffee.
	Strained fruit juice.
	Scrambled egg/boiled egg/grilled lean bacon/fish
	White bread—toasted (avoid wholemeal).
	Butter.
	Marmalade jelly—orange/lemon
	<div align="right">or honey/syrup.</div>
Mid-morning	Coffee.
Lunch	Meat/fish/omelette.
	Boiled potatoes—mashed.
	Sieved vegetables—peas/cabbage/beans/carrots/ turnips.
	Gravies/sauces.
	Sieved fruit/light sponge puddings/milk puddings —using ground grain, e.g. ground rice/jelly/.
Tea	White bread and butter or Hovis.
	Apple jelly/honey/syrup/blackcurrant jelly.
	Sponge cakes (free from dried fruit, cherries, peel, etc.).
Supper	Meat/fish/egg (avoid frying as a method of cooking).
	Creamed potato.
	Sieved vegetables—root or green.
	Jellies/sponges/moulds.

Bedtime   Milk drink—flavoured.

Foods not allowed—Salads, whole-grain cereals, breakfast cereals, whole fruit, dried fruit in cakes, fried foods, whole vegetables, nuts, seed jam, chunky marmalade.

The following foods would provide a daily intake of approximately 2000 Calories, suitable for a woman of 25 to 45 years in a sedentary occupation. It would also provide all the necessary foodstuffs in the correct proportions:

Meal	*Foods*
Breakfast	Cereal with milk and sugar.
	1 slice bread and butter/toast and marmalade.
	1 cup milky coffee.
Mid-morning	1 cup coffee.
	Sweet biscuit.
Lunch	Lamb chop/lean beef.
	Average helping potatoes and peas.
	Tinned fruit.
	Cheese and plain biscuits.
	Cup tea.
Tea	Cup tea.
	Sweet biscuit.
Supper	Ham omelette and tomato.
	2 slices bread and butter.
	Fresh fruit.
	1 cup milky coffee.
Bedtime	Milk drink.
	Sugar in drinks if liked.

The following foods would provide a daily intake of approximately 3200 Calories, suitable for a boy of 14. It would also provide all the necessary food factors in the correct proportions, with extra protein and carbohydrate, which is needed in this age group.

Meal	*Foods*
Breakfast	Breakfast cereal with milk and sugar.
	Egg and 2 rashers of bacon.
	3 slices bread and butter/toast and jam, honey or marmalade.
	Milk or milky coffee.
Mid-morning	⅓ pint milk.
	Cake/bun/slab chocolate.
Lunch	Large helping roast beef/stew/meat pie.
	Large helping potatoes and green vegetables.
	Sponge pudding/jam roll/apple pie.
	Apple/banana/orange.
Tea	Tea—2 cups.
	3 slices of bread and butter and jam.
	Cake/buns as desired.
Supper	Fried fish and chips.
	Tomato/vegetable.
	Fresh fruit.
	Cheese and biscuits.
	Milk or milky coffee.
Bedtime	Milk drink.
	Cake or biscuits.
	Apple.
	Sugar in drinks as desired.

References

Manual of Nutrition. (Ministry of Agriculture, Fisheries and Food), (1968). (London, Her Majesty's Stationery Office.)

HARRIS, C. F. (1963). *A Handbook of Dietetics for Nurses.* (London, Baillière, Tindall & Cassell Ltd.)

Chapter VI

OBSERVATIONS, EXAMINATIONS AND INVESTIGATIONS

The Oxford English Dictionary definition of observation includes the words "faculty of taking notice"; the ability to do this well depends on training and experience and is of particular importance in nursing. Although it is the medical staff who examine, diagnose and prescribe treatment, they rely on the nursing staff to observe and report on the changes in the patient's condition and behaviour throughout the 24 hours. In time, observation becomes a habit and, in fact, the clinical acumen of the experienced nurse is invaluable to the doctor.

How to observe.—The five senses provide the means by which information is acquired. They are sight, hearing, touch, smell and taste—the last named playing little part in clinical observation. As examples, the nurse may see changes in the patient's colour, may hear an alteration in his breathing, may feel a change in the rate and volume of his pulse and may smell a characteristic odour in his breath in certain conditions. At times she is asked to make specific observations, such as taking the temperature, pulse and respiration rates; at other times she may observe changes during the course of other duties—detailed care of the patient such as bathing in bed provide ideal opportunities. It is important to report accurately on what has been observed and not to draw conclusions.

Reporting.—Reports are made both verbally and in writing and both should be clear and concise. Verbal reports are made to the ward or night sister and through them to the doctor. Written reports differ in various hospitals, two main methods being in use:

1. A report book is kept on each ward, and detailed accounts are written of all new, or ill patients each evening by the ward sister, and early each morning by the senior night nurse. Copies or a précis of these may be sent to the central nursing office.

2. In the Kardex system the report is extremely brief, and is written on small cards, one of which is provided for each

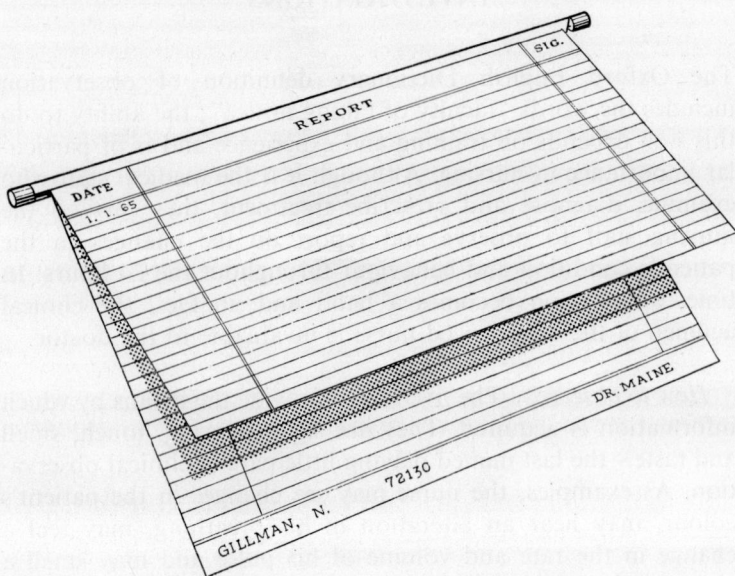

REPORT

DATE
1. 1. 65

SIG.

DR. MAINE

72130

GILLMAN, N.

FIG. 17.—"Kardex" (*Remington-Rand Ltd.*).

patient. This method saves time and is useful in that the patient's progress and treatment over several days can be seen at a glance. Where this system is used, a short report on the very ill patients may be sent to the central nursing office.

It is important in both systems that these reports are read by or given to all nurses when they come on duty, and that only abbreviations which are officially recognised should be used.

GENERAL OBSERVATIONS

Following admission, general observations are made on all patients, these include his colour, the appearance of skin and hair, his physique and any sign of recent loss of weight. It is possible to gain some idea as to whether the patient has any difficulty in seeing, hearing or walking, and to note the position he adopts when in bed. While carrying out bedside care the nurse may notice that certain movements are difficult for him.

During conversation a great deal may be learnt about the patient's background, previous illness, likes and dislikes, and worries. About 75% of those admitted to hospital adjust well, and have no particular emotional disturbance due to hospitalisation. The remaining 25% do not adapt to the new situation; this may show itself in many ways; for instance, a patient who is extremely frightened may be on the defensive and appear to resent and criticise all that is done for him. The fortunate 75% are often termed "good" patients; the remaining 25% are those who need greater sympathy and understanding, even if this is not well received.

TEMPERATURE, PULSE AND RESPIRATION RATES

Every patient in hospital has his temperature, pulse and respiration rates taken and recorded at regular intervals, as these three observations provide a guide to his condition and progress. The slang phrase in hospital "taking the temperatures" normally implies taking the pulse and respiration rates too. The intervals at which they are taken vary; for instance, in convalescent patients, once daily is enough—usually in the afternoon or early evening; for those in whom slight variations from normal may occur, a recording is made each morning and evening, and in the case of the very ill, every 4 hours.

Obviously in special circumstances it may be necessary to record one rate more frequently, without the other two; for example, the pulse may be taken every 15 or 30 minutes following major surgery.

Temperature

The normal range of body temperature (state of heat) is 36·1° to 37·3° C. (97° to 99° F.). The Fahrenheit (F.) scale is the one in common use in this country; on this the freezing point of

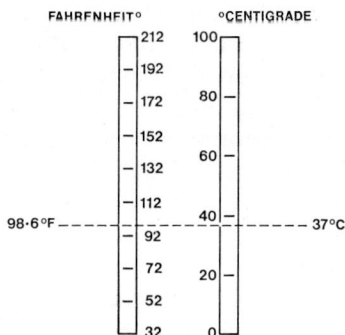

FIG. 18.—Comparison—Fahrenheit and Centigrade scales.

water is 32°, and the boiling point 212°. The Centigrade (C.) scale is gaining favour; on this the freezing point of water is 0 and the boiling point is 100. It will be seen from this that there are 100 divisions of the Centigrade scale between freezing and boiling points, and 180 in the Fahrenheit scale. The ratio is therefore $100:180 = 5:9$. To convert from Fahrenheit to Centigrade, 32 is subtracted, and the answer multiplied by $\frac{5}{9}$.

Example:

98·4° F. Normal body temperature.
$$98·4 - 32 = 66·4$$
$$\frac{66·4 \times 5}{9} = \frac{332}{9} = 36·8$$
36·8° C.

To convert from Centigrade to Fahrenheit the process is reversed ($\times \frac{9}{5} + 32$) but this is not often done.

It is necessary to use some instrument for an accurate measurement of temperature, since the skin (touch) is not a reliable guide. This instrument is the thermometer, the type varying according to function. The principle on which all thermometers are based is that on heating certain substances expand at a uniform rate, two examples being mercury and alcohol.

The clinical thermometer.—This is a mercury-filled thermometer designed for taking the body temperature; it is different from other thermometers in that there is a constriction between the bulb containing the mercury and the shaft. This thermometer is calibrated for a particular range—usually 35°–40° C., further subdivisions being to ·1°. A more definite mark is usually evident at 36·7° C., although, as mentioned, the normal range of temperature in health may be above or below this— in fact, being usually slightly higher in the evening than in the morning. The constriction is necessary to prevent the mercury returning to the bulb on removing the thermometer from the patient; once the level of the mercury has been noted and recorded, the thermometer is shaken to return it to the bulb.

Other thermometers (wall, lotion, bath, food).—These thermometers are larger, have a wider range, and have no constriction between the bulb and the shaft. It is important that these are read while the bulb is in the substance being tested, as the fluid level will drop (or rise) as soon as the bulb is removed.

Thermometers in common use in hospital are:

1. Clinical.
2. Wall.
3. Lotion, bath or food.

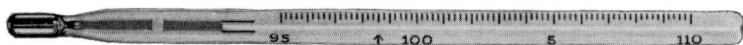

Fahrenheit

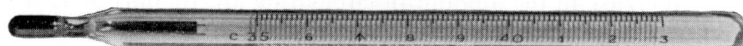

Celsius (or Centigrade)

Hypothermia (Subnormal)

Clinical Thermometers (*G. H. Zeal Ltd.*)

FIG. 19.—Thermometers.

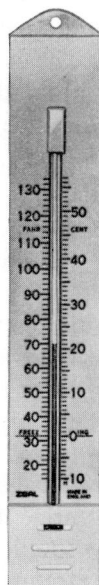

Wall Thermometer

Variations in temperature.—In health, the heat-regulating centre at the base of the brain controls the range of body temperature to a remarkable degree— the range being 1° C. in spite of great fluctuations in environmental conditions. Although small deviations from the normal are not necessarily serious, variations of approximately 5° C. either way are likely to be fatal, except in controlled conditions.

The most common cause of a rise in temperature (pyrexia) is infection—another being damage to the heat-regulating centre. The term hyper-pyrexia is used to describe very high temperatures, and since prolonged hyper-pyrexia can be dangerous, various measures are used to reduce the temperature. These include:

1. Removal of bedclothes.
2. Increase in the amount of circulating air, by fans or ventilation.
3. The use of ice compresses or ice bags.
4. Anti-pyretic drugs, e.g. aspirin.
5. Sponging with tepid water to increase evaporation from the skin and promote heat loss.

The term fever is also used to describe a rise in temperature and a patient with fever is described as being febrile.

The care of the febrile patient is the same, whatever the cause, and in addition to the normal basic nursing care it is important to remember the following:

As a result of the rise in temperature, the patient may well be hot and uncomfortable and may sweat more than usual. Frequent changes of clothing and bed linen and attention to the skin and mouth will be refreshing for him.

Because of the extra fluid loss, the salt and water balance is disturbed and the patient becomes very thirsty—and if fluid is not available, he may become dehydrated. Usually extra fluids by mouth will restore the balance. As a result of the pyrexia, the metabolic rate is increased and so more "fuel" is needed; for this reason extra glucose is often given —usually by being added to the fluid drunk. The patient's appetite will probably be poor, so a light, attractive diet should be offered and the patient encouraged to eat. Small frequent meals are often more acceptable. Another result of the extra fluid lost by the skin may be constipation, as there is less water available in the large bowel. Mild aperients or suppositories may be needed. It is common for the febrile patient to be restless and disorientated, and his sleep is often light and easily disturbed. All nursing measures to induce

82

sleep should be used as his need for rest is greater than normal.

Temperatures below 36·1° C. (97° F.) are described as being sub-normal. These occur as a defence mechanism whereby the body retains its heat, as a result of shock, haemorrhage, injury or operation. It must be emphasised that this is a normal reaction and it is unnecessary and often dangerous to apply artificial heat in an attempt to raise the temperature.

Hypothermia is the term used to describe a method whereby the temperature is deliberately lowered to several degrees below normal.

The pulse

The heart is a pump which, in the adult, contracts 60 to 80 times per minute; with each contraction (systole) blood is forced into the arteries which, because of their structure, are able to expand; during the resting phase of the heart (diastole) the arterial walls relax. This sequence of events can be felt at any point where an artery crosses a bone near to the surface of the body and is called the pulse. Much information about the circulatory system can be gained by regular observations on the rate, rhythm and volume of the pulse.

The rate varies with age, exercise, posture and emotion, and in disease. The infant has a pulse rate of 120 to 140 beats per minute, which gradually slows during childhood until the adult rate is reached; with advancing age the rate may be rather lower.

Exercise.—When normal rates are given it is assumed that the individual is awake, but at rest, the sleeping pulse rate being a little slower than normal. During exercise, the body's need for oxygen is greatly increased and the heart responds by beating more quickly. In the healthy person the rate returns to normal within a few minutes of resting. Many athletes and those "in training" have a normal pulse rate lower than the average.

Posture.—The rate is at its lowest when the subject is lying down, and slightly higher when sitting or standing, but these are very small variations.

Emotion.—Everyone is familiar with the fact that in times of stress or great pleasure the heart beats more strongly and more rapidly. Even during routine medical examinations doctors make allowance for this increase which may be the result of apprehension.

Disease.—It is not proposed to discuss specific illnesses, but obviously an increase or decrease in the normal pulse rate may be caused by disease. The most common examples of conditions associated with a raised pulse rate are haemorrhage—when the heart attempts to overcome the loss by pumping blood more quickly to the tissues; and when the temperature is raised—due to the increased metabolic rate. An example of a condition in which the pulse rate is abnormally slow is raised intracranial pressure. An increase in the heart rate is termed tachycardia, and a decrease, bradycardia.

Rhythm.—This is normally regular, and few variations occur except in illness. Occasionally a disturbance may be noted in that an extra beat occurs at irregular intervals; this is termed "extra systole" and commonly has no pathological significance; it may be noticed in those who are heavy smokers. With experience it will be possible for the nurse to distinguish between regular irregularities and irregular irregularities; in the former a recognisable pattern is repeated over and over again, and in the latter there is no pattern at all. The majority of irregularities in pulse rhythm are caused by some type of heart disease.

Volume.—To gain experience of the normal pulse volume the nurse is advised to take her own and her colleagues' pulses. The volume depends on the amount of circulating blood, the force of the heart beat and the state of the vessel walls. The volume is increased after exercise and in certain conditions affecting the lumen of the vessels; it is decreased following blood loss, shock and heart failure. The volume of the pulse gives some indication of the blood pressure, which will be discussed later.

Respiration

Breathing in is called inspiration and breathing out expiration; the two together being termed respiration. The normal respiration rate in the healthy adult is 16 to 20 times per minute, and breathing is quiet, regular and needs no conscious effort. Observations to be made include the rate and depth, and whether breathing is quiet or noisy, easy or difficult.

The rate.—This varies according to age, exercise, emotion and disease. The newborn baby breathes 35 to 40 times per minute, the rate slowing during early childhood; in the first few months of life breathing is often irregular.

Exercise and emotion.—As with the pulse, the rate is increased during exercise and in moments of stress.

Disease.—The respiratory rate is increased in many conditions —for example, in infections of the respiratory tract; it is decreased in some types of head injury and other conditions. As the metabolic rate rises in the febrile patient, so does the respiratory rate, and as it falls in hypothermia a similar fall in the breathing rate will be noted.

Certain drugs also depress the respiratory centre, so slowing the rate.

Depth.—The nurse will be familiar with the depth of normal breathing and will have noticed the difference following exercise. She will also notice variations in her patients' breathing—for example, respirations are shallow when the movements are painful and deep when the need for oxygen is increased.

Noise.—Noisy breathing may occur in the healthy person when asleep—snoring. In disease it is often due to some obstruction in the respiratory tract. The nurse should observe whether the noise is apparent on inspiration, expiration or both.

Dyspnoea, or difficult breathing, occurs in many conditions and is characterised by the use of muscles not normally used in breathing, e.g. the neck muscles, and by the fact that the patient is happier in a sitting position. The term apnoea is used to describe periods during which respirations are absent.

TAKING THE TEMPERATURE, PULSE AND RESPIRATION RATES

Before taking these rates it is important that the patient should have been at rest for a few minutes, in bed or in a chair, and that he has not recently had a hot or cold drink, or been smoking.

The most common place for taking the patient's temperature is in **the mouth**; the nurse makes sure that the mercury level is at 35° C., and places the thermometer under the patient's tongue; he should be asked to breathe through his nose.

While the thermometer is in position, the pulse and respiration rates are counted. The easiest place to feel the pulse is at the wrist, the nurse placing her fingers over the radial artery (thumb side). If at the same time the patient's arm is flexed across his chest, it will be possible, without any further movement, to count the respiration rate by noting the rise and fall of the chest. It is important that he does not become aware that the nurse is watching his breathing as the rate may increase. A watch with a clear second hand must be used. It is a common practice amongst nurses to "take the pulse" for 15 or 30 seconds and then multiply by 4 or 2 to obtain the minute rate; it is frequently quicker and always more accurate to count for a full minute. It is becoming increasingly common for the routine counting of respirations to be omitted except in the very ill; where this observation is required it must be accurate.

The thermometer is removed, the level of the mercury noted, the bulb wiped and the thermometer replaced in the container, which is commonly found on the wall at the head of the bed. Some mild antiseptic may be used in these containers.

The temperature, pulse and respiration rates are recorded on the patient's chart.

Thermometers should not be placed in the mouths of those who are:

1. Unconscious.
2. Mentally confused.
3. Very young.
4. Suffering from a blocked nose or a mouth infection.

Alternative sites for taking the temperature are the rectum and the groin or axilla.

The rectum.—The temperature here is slightly higher than in the mouth, so an indication must be made on the chart if the rectum is used. The end of the thermometer is lubricated with a little petroleum jelly and gently inserted a short distance into the anal canal. Babies and small children must be held firmly during this procedure. On removing the thermometer it is read, wiped and replaced as before.

The axilla and groin.—The temperature in these areas is slightly lower than that in the mouth, therefore an indication is made as above; it is important that the skin surfaces are dry and they must be in contact with the bulb of the thermometer. Three minutes should be allowed for the temperature to register.

When it is not practical to take the pulse at the wrist, it may be felt where an artery crosses a bone near the surface of the body. For example, at the temple, or just in front of the ear.

BLOOD PRESSURE

Blood pressure is the pressure exerted by the blood on the walls of the arteries, and is maintained by the volume and viscosity of circulating blood, the force of the heart beat, the capillary resistance and the elasticity of the vessel walls. In fact a pressure exists in the veins too (venous pressure), but the term "blood pressure" is normally taken to mean the pressure in the arteries and is commonly measured in the brachial artery. During systole, more blood enters the aorta, so causing a rise in pressure (systolic pressure), and during diastole the pressure falls (diastolic pressure).

Blood pressure is measured by an instrument called a sphygmomanometer, which consists of a tube containing mercury (Hg.) connected to an inflatable cuff; the tube is calibrated in millimeters. When air is pumped into the cuff the level of mercury rises. To take the blood pressure of a patient, the cuff is wound round the upper arm, and the tube connected to the sphygmomanometer; a stethoscope is placed over the brachial artery at the bend of the elbow, and the cuff is inflated until the pulse can no longer be felt at the wrist. The air is then slowly released and the level of the mercury watched; when the pressure in the cuff is just below that in the artery, blood will again flow down the vessel and sounds will be heard through the stethoscope. The level of the mercury is read at the first sound, this corresponding to the

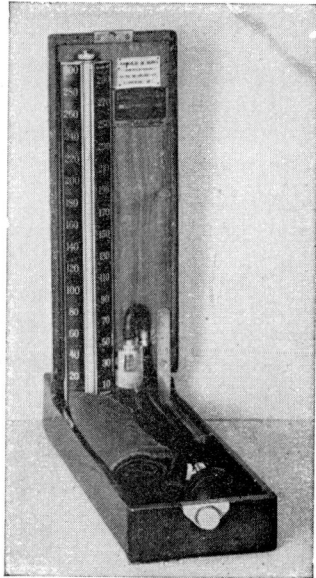

FIG. 20.—Sphygmomanometer.

systolic pressure; when the level is 30 to 40 mm. lower, the sounds will disappear, or alter in character; the reading at this point gives the diastolic pressure. Although it is easy to take the blood pressure of a healthy person, it is often difficult to hear the sounds in a patient who has collapsed or who has a low pressure.

The factors affecting blood pressure are age, exercise, posture, emotion and disease.

Age.—The blood pressure rises gradually throughout life—a rough guide to the normal systolic pressure in an adult being $110 + \frac{1}{2}$ age; the diastolic pressure is approximately 40 mm. lower.

Exercise, posture and emotion.—These affect the systolic pressure in the same way as the pulse, and it is therefore just as important to have the patient at rest for a few minutes before taking it.

Disease.—Many diseases affect the blood pressure; some make it higher, e.g. hardening of the arteries and some kidney disorders; and a low blood pressure is noticed in conditions such as shock and haemorrhage.

Recording of the blood pressure. This is recorded as follows:

$$\text{B.P.} = \frac{\text{Systolic pressure}}{\text{Diastolic pressure}} \text{ mm./Hg.}$$

Although the taking of blood pressure is a frequent observation and often of great importance, it is possible to obtain much information about the patient's condition without using a sphygmomanometer.

THE SKIN

The skin is the epithelial covering of the body and is normally supple, elastic and dry and warm to the touch.

Variations which may occur are:

(a) The skin may be excessively dry and inelastic. This is present in patients who are dehydrated, and therefore in those who have prolonged pyrexia. Lack of elasticity occurs normally in the elderly.

(b) Excessive sweating. This obviously occurs after exercise, especially in the areas where sweat glands are numerous, but in certain conditions such as shock the nurse may notice that the whole skin feels clammy.

(c) Small superficial harmorrhages may occur into the skin; these are known as petechiae, or purpura, and are the result of a defect in the blood-clotting mechanism.

(d) Rashes are characteristic of many conditions, particularly the infectious fevers of childhood, e.g. measles, and in allergies.

(e) Changes due to specific skin diseases, e.g. eczema; in these the skin may be moist, with "weeping" areas, or excessively dry and scaly.

Colour

Variations in colour are as follows:

(a) Pallor. This occurs in shock, haemorrhage, and also if the patient is anaemic.

(b) Cyanosis. This term is used to describe blueness of the skin and mucous membranes. It may be seen in patients with an obstructed airway and those with certain types of heart disease.

(c) Jaundice, or yellowness of the skin and mucous membranes, is due to the presence of excess bile pigments in the blood, and occurs in many conditions affecting the liver and biliary apparatus. It may also be present as a result of excessive breakdown of red blood cells, e.g. after an incompatible transfusion.

(d) The term "flushed" is used to describe a high colour which may be due to a high temperature, high blood pressure or other conditions.

COUGH

This is a normal defence mechanism which occurs when the respiratory tract is irritated, and helps to dislodge and expel the irritant. The reflex centre concerned is situated in the brain stem and is to a certain extent under voluntary control; it may be depressed by drugs and anaesthetic substances. A cough is described as being:

(a) Dry, or unproductive, when no sputum is produced; this occurs in the early stages of respiratory infection and in heavy smokers, and is sometimes "nervous" in origin.

(b) Productive cough is one where sputum is produced and occurs in many respiratory conditions. In these cases the patient should expectorate into a waxed carton which is burnt after use. The sputum is measured (in the carton) and a report made on the amount and type; it may be described as being thin and watery, thick and purulent, or sometimes bloodstained. The coughing up of blood is termed haemoptysis.

VOMIT

When a patient is sick, the term vomit is used to describe the material ejected from the stomach. This may contain undigested food, bile or blood; vomiting blood is called haematemesis. The causes of vomiting are numerous and include food poisoning, obstruction of the digestive tract, certain drugs and anaesthetic substances, and stress. Observations are made on the amount, colour, contents and smell; and also the relationship to pain, food and movement.

FAECES

Faeces are a normal waste product excreted from the rectum. In health, a few grammes of semi-solid brown material with a characteristic odour are passed daily.

Abnormalities, which may be observed, include:

(a) Fresh blood; this denotes some lesion in the lower bowel.
(b) Digested blood; the faeces appear black and tarry (melaena); this occurs when blood is swallowed, or there is bleeding from the stomach and the small intestine.
(c) Foreign bodies; this is reasonably common in young children who tend to swallow small objects.
(d) Intestinal worms; various worms, e.g. threadworms, may be seen in the stools when infestation is present.
(e) Changes in colour; in biliary obstruction, no bile pigments reach the intestine and the faeces are pale and putty coloured; in acute intestinal infections (especially in babies) the faeces may be fluid and green; changes also occur due to drugs, e.g. iron, which make the stools black.

URINE

Normal urine is pale yellow in colour and has a specific gravity of 1·010 to 1·025. Its composition is:

Water 96%   Urea 2%   Salts 2%

It is normally slightly acid in reaction.

When the fluid intake is less than usual, or when there is

excessive sweating, vomiting or diarrhoea, the amount of urine is reduced, it is darker in colour (concentrated), and the specific gravity is high. When the fluid intake is increased, and in cold weather, the amount of urine is greater, the colour is paler (dilute) and the specific gravity is nearer to that of water.

The following terms are used:

(a) Polyuria: an increase in the amount of urine passed.
(b) Oliguria: a great decrease in the amount of urine passed.
(c) Anuria: less than 60 mls. of urine passed per day.
(d) Dysuria: pain or difficulty on micturition.
(e) Haematuria: the presence of blood in the urine.
(f) Retention: urine is secreted by the kidneys, but retained in the bladder due to obstruction or nerve injury.
(g) Suppression: failure of the kidneys to secrete urine.

Changes in colour occur:

(a) In jaundice—when bile pigments appear in the urine, making it greenish-brown.
(b) When certain drugs or foods are taken.
(c) In haematuria.

In infections of the urinary tract, the urine appears cloudy and commonly has an unpleasant smell.

Many abnormal substances may be present in urine in disease: some of these are visible to the naked eye, e.g. blood and bile; others are found when the urine is tested in the ward or laboratory. Ward tests are simple but need to be carried out efficiently and the results reported accurately; errors in ward testing are commonly due to dirty equipment, old (stale) reagents, or perhaps lack of understanding by the nurse. In recent years, tablets and impregnated "strips" have replaced the numerous liquid reagents in many hospitals. The advantages of the newer tests are speed and simplicity, and provided the maker's instructions are followed, it is difficult to make a mistake. The older tests may be preferred and in some cases are thought to be more accurate.

All urine should be tested using clean equipment; the reaction should be taken using litmus paper (blue paper turning red = acid), and the specific gravity found using a urinometer.

Ward tests may be carried out to establish the presence or absence of albumin (protein), sugar, ketones—acetone and diacetic acid—or blood.

Reagents   **Tablet or strip**

ALBUMIN

1. *Cold test.*—One inch of urine is placed in a test tube; 5 drops of salicyl sulphonic acid are added; if albumin is present, a white cloud appears.

   Albustix.—Dip the impregnated end of the stick in the urine; note any colour change, and compare with the colour chart provided.

2. *Hot test.*—A test tube is $\frac{2}{3}$ filled with urine; the upper $\frac{1}{3}$ is boiled; if a cloud forms, a few drops of acetic acid are added; if the cloud is still present, the test is positive.

3. *Esbach's quantitative test.*—A specimen from a 24-hour collection is used; the urine must be acid (if not, add acetic acid), and the specific gravity must be 1·010 or less (if it is higher—dilute with water using known quantities).

   Fill the graduated Esbach's tube with urine up to the letter U, and with Esbach's reagent up to the letter R: stand for 24 hours. The level of the white deposit is read as the number of grammes of albumin per litre of urine; (if the urine was diluted, the figure must now be multiplied to obtain the correct result).

SUGAR

Benedict's test.—Five mls. of Benedict's solution (copper sulphate) is placed in a test tube, and 8 to 10 drops of urine are added; the test tube is heated gently and the fluid boiled; any colour change is noted and reported, and will indicate the amount of sugar present;

Clinistix.—This merely indicates the presence or absence of glucose; the impregnated end of the strip is dipped in the urine, and compared with the colour chart.

92

colour changes may be green—yellow—orange—brick red.

Clinitest.—This is a quantitative test; 5 drops of urine and 10 drops of water are placed in a test tube; 1 tablet is added; when the effervescence has stopped, the colour is compared with a chart.

ACETONE

Rothera's test.—Two inches of urine are placed in a test tube and saturated with ammonium sulphate and sodium nitroprusside crystals (Rothera's crystals); ½ inch of strong ammonia is added; if acetone is present, a violet ring appears.

Acetest.—A tablet is placed on a white tile and 1 drop of urine is added; after 30 seconds the colour is compared with a chart.

DIACETIC ACID
(Aceto-acetic acid)

One inch of urine is placed in a test tube; ferric chloride solution is added slowly; if deep red colour appears, either salicylates or diacetic acid are present; boil the solution; if the colour disappears, diacetic acid is present, and acetone must also be present.

No test.

BLOOD

If this is not visible to the naked eye, then laboratory tests are needed.

Occultest.—One drop of urine is placed on a filter paper, and a tablet placed in the centre; 2 drops of water are placed on the tablet; if a blue colour appears on the paper within 2 minutes, the test is positive.

INTAKE AND OUTPUT (FLUID BALANCE) CHARTS

It is often necessary to know whether a patient's fluid intake is satisfactory and whether the intake and output balance. On paper, it is rarely possible to equate all types of fluid gained and lost; for example, it is difficult to assess the water produced during metabolism, or the water lost in perspiration. However, the fluid drunk and the urine passed will give some indication of the fluid balance. At times the following may also be recorded —intravenous, rectal or subcutaneous fluids (intake), and vomit, gastric aspiration or drainage (output). These observations must be accurately recorded on the appropriate chart, the metric system—litres and millilitres—is used as the scale of measurement.

EXAMINATION OF THE PATIENT

All patients are examined by the doctor shortly after admission, and the nurse is often present to assist him. This examination is a complete physical "check-up" to provide a clinical picture of the patient's condition. It is important that the patient is relaxed and co-operative, and to achieve this the nurse should prepare him beforehand by explaining who the doctor is, and his connection with other medical staff whom the patient may have seen earlier. During the examination privacy is essential, and he should be exposed as little as possible.

The order of the examination may vary and the following is merely a guide to the patient's position and the equipment which may be needed.

Examination of the chest and abdomen

The patient will be examined alternately lying flat and sitting up; and the doctor uses three methods:

1. **Percussion.**—This is a way of obtaining information about various organs, e.g. the lungs, by tapping with the fingers and observing the sound produced.

2. **Palpation.**—Organs which are easily felt may be examined by gentle pressure of the hand, and irregularities, such as hardness or enlargement, noted.

3. **Auscultation.**—This term is derived from the Latin "ausculto"—to listen, and is normally carried out with a stethoscope; the doctor generally provides his own.

Examination of the eyes and ears.—The patient should be in a comfortable position, either sitting up or lying down. Much information may already have been gained by the nurse regarding the patient's sight and hearing, and wherever difficulties are observed these should be reported. For detailed information a careful examination is necessary:

The eyes: the patient's accommodation to light is tested using a small torch, and the retina examined with an ophthalmoscope.

The ears are examined using an auroscope—this has a detachable speculum, which should be cleaned and sterilized after use.

Examination of body cavities

1. **Mouth and throat.**—To examine these the doctor will need a good light and a tongue depressor; if a wooden spatula is used, it is discarded after use; if metal, it is washed and sterilised. Post-nasal or laryngeal mirrors may be required.

2. **Rectal examination (P.R.).**—This is not always carried out, but is a relatively common examination; the patient should lie in the left lateral position with the knees drawn up. The doctor examines the rectum with a gloved finger; if a lubricant is required, either petroleum jelly or K.Y. jelly is satisfactory. Disposable finger cots or stalls are thrown away after use; should rubber gloves be used for this procedure they must be washed and sterilised before being used again. Many wards keep a rectal tray available for immediate use.

Examination of the central nervous system

During routine examination certain reflexes are tested, e.g. the knee jerk; for these a patella hammer is used. Should any abnormality be found, a more detailed examination is carried out to test the special senses (sight, hearing, smell and taste) and to observe the reaction to light and deep touch, pain, heat and cold. The following equipment may be required: ophthalmoscope, auroscope, tuning fork, liquids with a strong smell, e.g. peppermint, salt and sugar, cotton wool, pins, test tubes with hot and cold water, a pencil torch, spatulae, a tape measure (to test for muscle wasting), a skin pencil and a container for used equipment.

INVESTIGATIONS

Having examined the patient, the doctor may order certain investigations to be carried out during his stay in hospital. These include examination of specimens of blood and secretions and excretions, and X-rays of various parts of the body.

Collection of specimens

1. **Urine.**—These may be routine specimens,
                    clean specimens,
                    catheter specimens.

(a) Routine specimens are collected for ward testing and occasionally to go to the laboratory. They require no preparation of the patient, are usually collected early in the morning, and are transferred from the bedpan or urinal to a clean container which is labelled with the date, patient's name and the time of collection.

(b) Clean specimens: as the name implies, everything connected with this specimen is clean; the patient, the receptacle into which the urine is passed and the container. If the patient is allowed up, he can wash the area around the urethra before passing urine. If confined to bed, the area is cleansed using a suitable lotion and wool swabs. In the male patient a mid-stream specimen is obtained, the patient starting to pass urine into a urinal and then collecting the subsequent urine into a clean receptacle. This technique may be applied to women but unless special tubes are available it presents certain practical difficulties. A clean specimen is obtained when bacteriological tests are necessary; these are carried out in the laboratory. It is replacing the catheter specimen wherever possible, as the latter carries the risk of introducing infection into the urinary tract.

(c) Catheter specimens. This is an aseptic procedure and will be discussed later (see page 150).

2. **Faeces.**—It is important that a specimen of faeces is fresh; a small amount is removed from the bedpan, using a wooden spatula, and is placed in a waxed carton; the wooden spatula is discarded. In certain cases it may be necessary to send the

whole specimen, and in this situation the bedpan is simply covered and taken at once to the laboratory.

3. **Sputum.**—This is best obtained first thing in the morning as the patient is most likely to produce sputum at this time, secretions having collected in the respiratory tract during the night. He is given a container and asked to expectorate; clear instructions are important as sputum is required and not saliva.

4. **Blood.**—Blood specimens are required for numerous investigations, and in varying quantities. The blood is taken from the patient either by a laboratory technician or a doctor; the amounts required range from a few drops squeezed from a pricked finger, to 10 mls. taken from a vein in the arm.

Various tubes are used to receive the specimen; they fall into 2 main groups:

(a) Those containing no chemical—often called "plain" or "universal" tubes. They are used when serum is required for the test as the blood will clot, and separate into the solid clot (cells) and the liquid (serum).

(b) Those containing some substance which prevents the blood from clotting; this may be a salt such as oxalate or citrate, or an organic substance such as heparin. These are used when tests on whole blood are required.

The nurse should explain the procedure to the patient, provide the doctor with equipment, e.g. a sterile syringe, swabs, lotion and a container, and assist him if necessary. If a needle is inserted into a vein, the procedure is called venupuncture. Following the taking of blood, a swab is placed over the puncture for a few minutes; the nurse should see that the patient is comfortable.

5. **Swabs.**—Specimens of material may be taken from any moist surface of the body, e.g. throat, skin, vagina, to determine the presence or absence of pathogenic organisms. Sterile dressed orange sticks are used and obtained from the laboratory. It is essential that the nurse has a good light, and that the patient understands what she is about to do, especially in the case of a throat swab. When taking a swab from the inside of a body cavity, it may be necessary to use a speculum to avoid touching

other parts; for the throat a tongue depressor is used. On completion, the orange stick is returned to its container and sent to the laboratory.

All specimens for the laboratory must be carefully labelled with the patient's name, the ward, the date and time of collection. They are taken by a messenger, with the appropriate request form signed by a doctor as soon as they are obtained. Containers having screw tops must be firmly closed to avoid contamination of other specimens or forms.

X-rays.—An X-ray picture is a common aid to diagnosis; it is similar to a photograph, but the short waves used pass through soft tissues and show up denser tissues, fluid and air. If a picture of soft tissue is needed, some contrast medium is introduced into the body to outline or fill the part under examination. The contrast media used are:

(1) Barium sulphate—this is non-toxic and is not absorbed.

(2) Various iodine compounds, e.g. Diodone or Lipiodol.

(3) Air.

The preparation of the patient is important and varies according to the part being X-rayed. It is essential that the area should not be obscured by metal fastenings, hair pins or buttons; for this reason, most patients are undressed and given a simple open-backed gown fastened with tapes.

Straight X-ray

This is a picture taken without the use of contrast media and can be used for any part of the body. It is a common procedure for suspected fractures, or in routine examination of the chest.

X-rays of the digestive tract

(a) Barium swallow, meal, and follow through. The patient is given nothing to eat or drink for at least 4 hours beforehand; in the X-ray department he is given a glass of barium sulphate solution to drink and pictures are taken at intervals. These outline the oesophagus, stomach and small intestine; the barium is later passed in the faeces, which are therefore grey in colour.

(b) Barium enema. The preparation includes the emptying of the lower bowel, which is usually achieved by the use of Dulcolax suppositories. In the department, a solution of barium sulphate is introduced into the rectum (see page 142) and pictures are taken. This outlines the large intestine.

X-rays of the urinary tract

As the kidneys and ureters are situated at the back of the abdominal cavity, it is important that as little air as possible is present in the intestine, as this will cast shadows and obscure the outline. This is usually no problem if the patient is up and about, but in certain cases substances which absorb air, e.g. charcoal, may be given by mouth the night before the X-ray.

(a) Intravenous pyelogram. An iodine compound is injected intravenously; this will be carried in the blood stream to the kidneys and excreted in the urine. If pictures are taken at this point, an outline of the urinary tract will be seen. It is customary to restrict the fluid intake for 4 hours beforehand, in order to concentrate the urine.

(b) Retrograde pyelogram. The patient is prepared as for a general anaesthetic (page 174). In the theatre, an instrument (catheterising cystoscope) is passed into the bladder, per urethrum, and fine catheters introduced into the ureters. Through these an iodine compound is injected into the pelvis of the kidney; X-ray pictures are then taken, these outline the pelvis, ureters, bladder and, in some cases, the urethra.

X-rays of the biliary apparatus

Cholecystogram. The evening before the X-ray a light, fat-free meal is given; 12 hours before the X-ray the medium is given. This is supplied by the department in the form of a powder which is dissolved in water or fruit juice. No further food, fluids or drugs are given until after the first pictures have been taken.

X-rays of the circulatory system

It is possible to outline the blood supply to a part by injecting an iodine compound into the artery supplying the organ (arteriogram) or, in the case of the heart, into a vein returning blood from the systemic circulation (angio-cardiogram). The preparations vary, and details are normally prescribed for each patient.

X-rays of the bronchial tree

A bronchogram is an introduction of an iodised oil into the trachea, either via the mouth, or by an injection in the neck. The patient is then moved into different positions so that the medium reaches all lobes of both lungs; pictures are then taken. The preparation of the patient is as for a general anaesthetic, and the after-care is important as the back of the throat will be insensitive for several hours and the patient must not eat or drink. Later he is encouraged to cough up the oil.

X-rays of the ventricles of the brain

In ventriculography and air-encephelography, air is the contrast medium; as its introduction involves either a lumbar puncture, or surgery, it will be discussed later.

It is the custom in many X-ray departments to carry out skin tests on patients before an iodine medium is used; this limits the risk of severe allergic reactions.

Medicines may be omitted for 24 hours before any X-ray involving contrast media.

All patients going to the X-ray department should be warmly clad, and the nurse must see that they are comfortable if a long waiting period seems likely. When the patient returns from the department, enquiries should be made as to when he may eat or drink.

Chapter VII

ANTISEPSIS AND ASEPSIS

Infection has been a problem in hospitals for many hundreds of years. During the 18th and 19th centuries, various discoveries led to a great increase in understanding the causes of infection and many famous men evolved techniques which lowered the incidence and reduced the mortality rate.

The foundation stone of bacteriology was the invention of the microscope, when for the first time minute living organisms were seen in water, soil and scrapings from human tissue. Even before it was realised that these organisms could cause disease, Semmelweiss taught his students to wash their hands between carrying out post-mortems on patients who had died from infection and delivering women in labour, thus greatly reducing the numbers of mothers and babies who died from sepsis. Later Pasteur linked organisms with specific diseases, and he was followed by many others who developed ways of identifying and classifying bacteria, and methods of preventing infection by the use of antiseptics.

In the last 30 years the discovery of the sulphonamide drugs and the newer antibiotic substances, together with the development of aseptic techniques, led to advances in surgery thought to be impossible before, and to a belief that hospital infection was conquered. However, the ability of certain organisms to develop a resistance to modern drugs has created a problem of no less magnitude than that of the pre-antibiotic era.

Antisepsis is the technique of killing bacteria present by the use of chemicals.

Asepsis, on the other hand, implies that all articles are rendered sterile before being used, so that infection should not occur.

Sterilisation means rendering an article free from living micro-organisms. It is important for the nurse to realise that a thing is either sterile or unsterile and that there are no half measures or "almost sterile" techniques.

101

METHODS OF STERILISATION

1. Heat

(a) Dry heat

An article will be sterile if kept at a temperature of 160° C. for 1 hour (320° F.).

The apparatus used for this is a hot-air oven, which works on the same principle as the domestic oven.

This method is suitable for all glass, stainless steel or enamel ware and has the advantage that equipment can be sterilised assembled, i.e. syringe with needle fitted in a container—so that it is ready for immediate use.

If dressings are to be sterilised by dry heat, a lower temperature and a longer time are necessary, otherwise discoloration and charring will result.

(b) Moist heat

Boiling

This is a common but rather unsatisfactory method of sterilising equipment in hospital wards. Its advantages are its simplicity and speed—5 minutes' boiling will kill all bacteria. Its disadvantages are that spores are not affected by boiling, and often faults in technique lead to articles being used which have not been properly sterilised.

To be effective the following points must be observed:

(i) The articles must be clean before being placed in the steriliser.

(ii) The water must completely cover all articles, which should be placed separately, and not "stacked".

(iii) The timing must not start until the water is actually boiling, and from this point no further articles must be placed in the steriliser; it is this last point which is so difficult to supervise adequately in a busy ward.

(iv) When sterilisation is complete the articles must be removed, using sterile forceps which are kept for this purpose—Cheatle or bowl forceps.

This method is still used to sterilise ward equipment in many hospitals, e.g. instruments, bowls, receivers and occasionally syringes.

The Autoclave

This is a method of sterilisation using steam under pressure; the increased pressure has the effect of raising the temperature of the steam above boiling point, as shown below:

5 lb. pressure 109° C.
10 lb.   ,,   115° C.
15 lb.   ,,   121° C.
20 lb.   ,,   126° C.
32 lb.   ,,   134° C.

As the temperature is higher, both bacteria and spores are killed, and because of this the autoclave is a more efficient method of sterilisation than boiling.

An autoclave works on the same principle as the domestic pressure cooker: in both, the container is closed, the temperature raised, air driven out and the compartment filled with steam. At this point the vent through which the air has been escaping is closed and heating continues, so increasing the pressure within the container. When the desired pressure is reached, the controls of the autoclave are set to maintain this for the time necessary to sterilise the enclosed articles. At the end of this time steam is replaced by hot air which dries the contents, and when the pressure returns to normal the autoclave is opened and the articles are ready for use.

The above merely describes the principle on which most autoclaves work, and in fact modern machines are complex and are automatically controlled.

The size of the autoclave varies. Small ones are now being fitted in some wards to replace the steriliser, and large units are used in theatres and central departments.

Almost all hospital equipment can be sterilised by this method, the pressure and time being altered according to the material of which the article is made. For example, rubber articles may be sterilised at a lower pressure than ward dressings, and for a shorter time.

It is important that steam is able to penetrate to all parts of the article; for this reason syringes and other equipment must not be assembled, and dressings must be packed loosely in their container—e.g. metal drum with perforated sides, or a paper, cardboard or other pack.

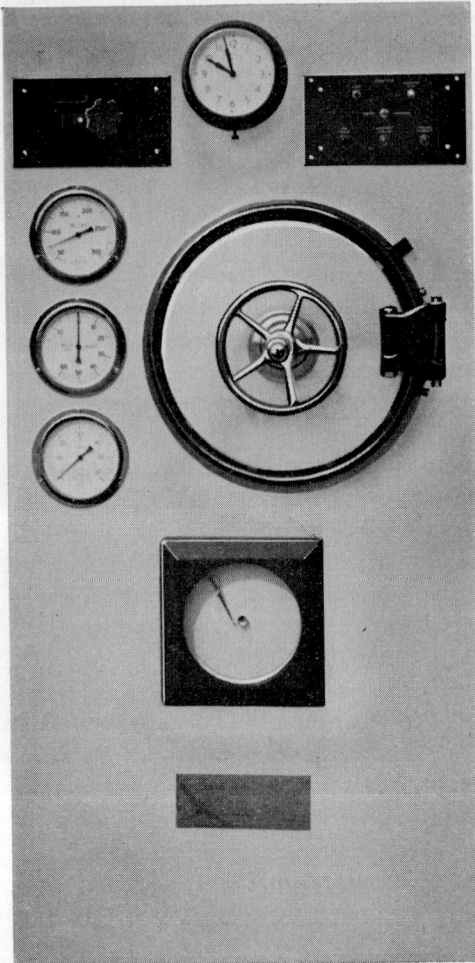

FIG. 21.—A Modern Autoclave (*Down Bros.*).

Various devices are used to test the efficiency of the autoclave. Briefly, these consist of impregnated paper strips, or tubes, which change colour if the correct temperature is reached. These are incorporated in the outer part of a pack or placed in the centre of a drum.

104

2. Chemicals

Since Lister's use of carbolic acid sprays as a means of reducing infection, a large number of antiseptics and disinfectants have been introduced for a wide range of uses. The terms "disinfectant" and "antiseptic" are loosely used both inside and outside hospital, and far too much faith is placed in their efficacy.

To be efficient certain conditions must be fulfilled:

(i) The correct strength must be used.
(ii) The article must be clean and free from blood and pus.
(iii) The article must be completely immersed in the solution.
(iv) The two must be in contact for a given length of time.

It is rather more common to use chemicals to disinfect articles that have been contaminated, before returning them to general use, than to use them to sterilise articles required for aseptic techniques.

Ethylene oxide gas

This may be used for the sterilisation of heat labile products, plastics, respirator components etc.

Lotions in common use

The lotions in use in hospitals today are so numerous that it is impossible to do more than give a few examples. For detailed descriptions the nurse is advised to read a textbook of bacteriology, and to refer to her hospital procedure book for local practice.

(a) A large group of disinfectants are the **phenols and cresols** (coal tar derivatives); these include carbolic acid, lysol and Sudol. All are irritating to human tissue and are used for disinfecting or sterilising metal instruments and excreta. Sudol is less irritating than lysol or phenol, but even so it is advisable to wear gloves when using any of these. Articles disinfected in this way need to be rinsed thoroughly in water before use. Chloroxylenols (e.g. Dettol) are similar to the phenols, but are much less toxic.

(b) **The Halogens.** This group includes iodine, chlorine and its derivatives, such as the hypochlorites (Milton). Iodine may be used on the skin in weak solution. It is appropriate to point out here that it is impossible to sterilise the skin; any solution strong enough to destroy all bacteria would completely destroy the tissue. Hypochlorites may be used to disinfect glassware such as urinals, or babies' feeding bottles, or plastic equipment that will not stand boiling. It is not essential to rinse the article after using these solutions.

(c) **Soapy solutions** such as Hycolin, Roccal or Bradasol are particularly useful as cleansing agents. Since these are non-toxic they can be used on the skin and help to remove grease and dirt.

(d) **Chlorhexidine** (Hibitane) may be used for sterilising sharp instruments, 0.5% in 70% spirit: it can also be applied to the skin and used for irrigation purposes—aqueous solution 1 in 5000.

(e) Other groups of antiseptics include the **dyes**—e.g. gentian violet, **the alcohols**—e.g. methylated spirit, and **the oxidising agents**—e.g. hydrogen peroxide.

Except where actual sterilisation is required, or a specific infection is present, the best cleansing solution for either the skin or inanimate objects is hot, soapy water. Both patients and staff are often happier when an "antiseptic smell" is present.

Dilution of lotions.—The importance of using the correct strength of a lotion has already been mentioned; should this strength not be available, a stronger solution may be diluted. The following formula is applicable:

$$\frac{\text{Strength of solution available}}{\text{Strength of solution required}} = \text{Proportion of strong solution required in total amount; the rest is water.}$$

Example

600 mls. of 1 in 80 Sudol required.

Solution available: 1 in 20 Sudol.

$$\frac{1 \text{ in } 20}{1 \text{ in } 80} = \frac{1}{4}$$

106

$\frac{1}{4}$ of 600 mls. (150 mls) of 1 in 20 Sudol.

$+$

$\frac{3}{4}$ of 600 mls. (450 mls.) of water = 600 mls. of 1 in 80 Sudol.

3. Irradiation

It is possible to sterilise some hospital equipment, e.g. syringes, by using infra red rays. The unit is expensive to install, but the process of sterilisation with this method is quick, in some instances taking only a few minutes. Much of the pre-sterilised disposable equipment now in use—for example, syringes and catheters—is sterilised by gamma radiation.

DISPOSABLES

The use of disposable equipment has greatly increased over the last few years, and has the advantages of lessening the risk of cross-infection and saving time. These items are made of in-expensive materials and include:

Paper—replacing cloth.
>	Examples: masks, bedpan covers, clinical sheets (dressing towels), nurses caps and hand towels.

Plastics—replacing glass, rubber and, more recently, metal.
>	Examples: syringes, catheters and various tubes, oxygen masks, and blood-transfusion sets, dissecting forceps and scalpels.

Tin foil—replacing stainless steel or enamel ware.
>	Examples: gallipots and instruments trays.

The disposal of these articles after use has created certain problems, particularly where plastics are concerned, as these do not burn in all types of furnace. The cost is also a matter for concern, but with increasing use the prices may fall, and obviously the use of disposable equipment has meant a reduction in laundry and labour costs.

CENTRAL STERILE SUPPLY DEPARTMENT (C.S.S.D.)

Recent surveys have shown that methods of sterilisation in hospital wards leave much to be desired; also a great deal of time is spent by the nursing staff in packing drums, setting and clearing away trays and trolleys, and in caring for equipment.

For these and many other reasons Central Sterile Supply Departments are planned for new hospitals and are being set up in many existing hospitals. The idea of these central departments is that they shall supply sterile equipment for procedures to all wards and departments, and be responsible for the cleansing of such equipment after use.

The size of these departments varies greatly, some being designed and built for the purpose, others being started in one

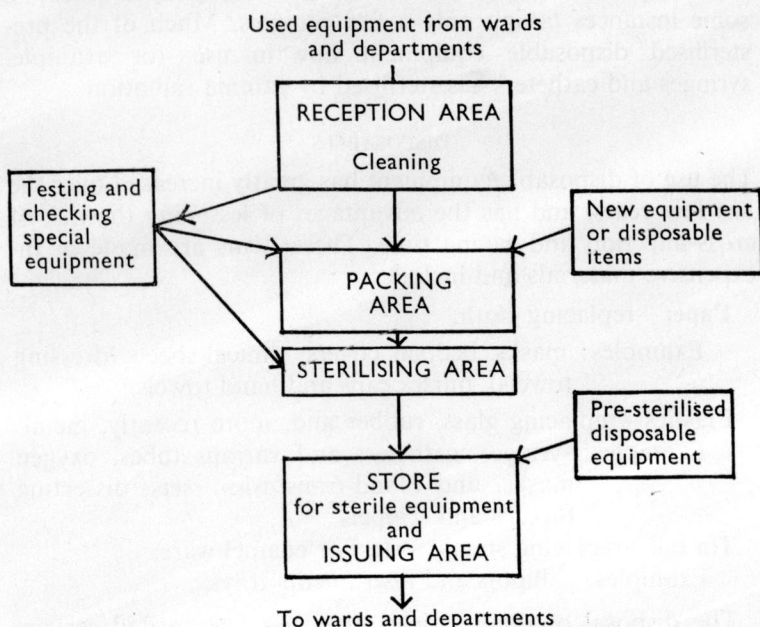

Used equipment from wards
and departments

RECEPTION AREA

Cleaning

Testing and
checking
special
equipment

New equipment
or disposable
items

PACKING
AREA

STERILISING AREA

Pre-sterilised
disposable
equipment

STORE
for sterile equipment
and
ISSUING AREA

To wards and departments

PLAN OF A CENTRAL STERILE SUPPLY DEPARTMENT

Fig. 22

or two existing rooms. The scope depends on size and sterilising equipment available, some departments merely providing a central syringe service.

As this is relatively a new idea, there is as yet no fixed pattern of staffing, but some of the present C.S.S.D.'s are supervised by an experienced nurse, who may be responsible to the matron, the pharmacist or the bacteriologist. The tendency seems to be to employ non-nursing personnel to staff the department,

although student nurses may spend 1 to 2 weeks
of their training as observers.

The contents of the packs supplied vary fro
hospital, but the principle in all cases is that for
cedure a fresh pack (or packs) is opened and mat
is returned for re-sterilisation. Disposable equipment is often
incorporated, and after use is discarded.

The contents of a small dressing pack might be as follows:

4 wool swabs.	1 or 2 clinical sheets.
4 gauze swabs.	1 (tinfoil) gallipot.
4 pairs forceps.	

These would be wrapped firstly in a clinical sheet which will
later serve as a sterile surface, and secondly in a protective
covering which may be a paper bag, paper sheeting, cellophane
or balloon cloth.

Methods of distribution vary but it should not be necessary
to keep large stocks on individual wards.

Many hospitals without a C.S.S.D. are using commercial
dressing packs prepared by various firms, rather than sterilising
their own dressings in metal drums.

CROSS-INFECTION

The term "cross-infection" implies that a patient acquires an
infection in hospital which he did not have when he was admitted. The diagram below indicates the ways by which infection may be spread.

This type of infection is a serious matter, since it occurs in
someone who is already sick and delays recovery, so prolonging
his stay in hospital. Since antibiotics are widely used, it may
well be caused by resistant bacteria and therefore be difficult to
treat. It may show itself in a number of ways, and although
wound infection in a surgical ward is an obvious example,
throat and urinary infections can also occur in any ward. In
children's wards measles and gastro-enteritis are examples of
infections which may spread from one child to another.

Methods of prevention

The ward plan.—It is obviously easier to prevent infection in
a small unit than in a large open ward; the spacing of beds is

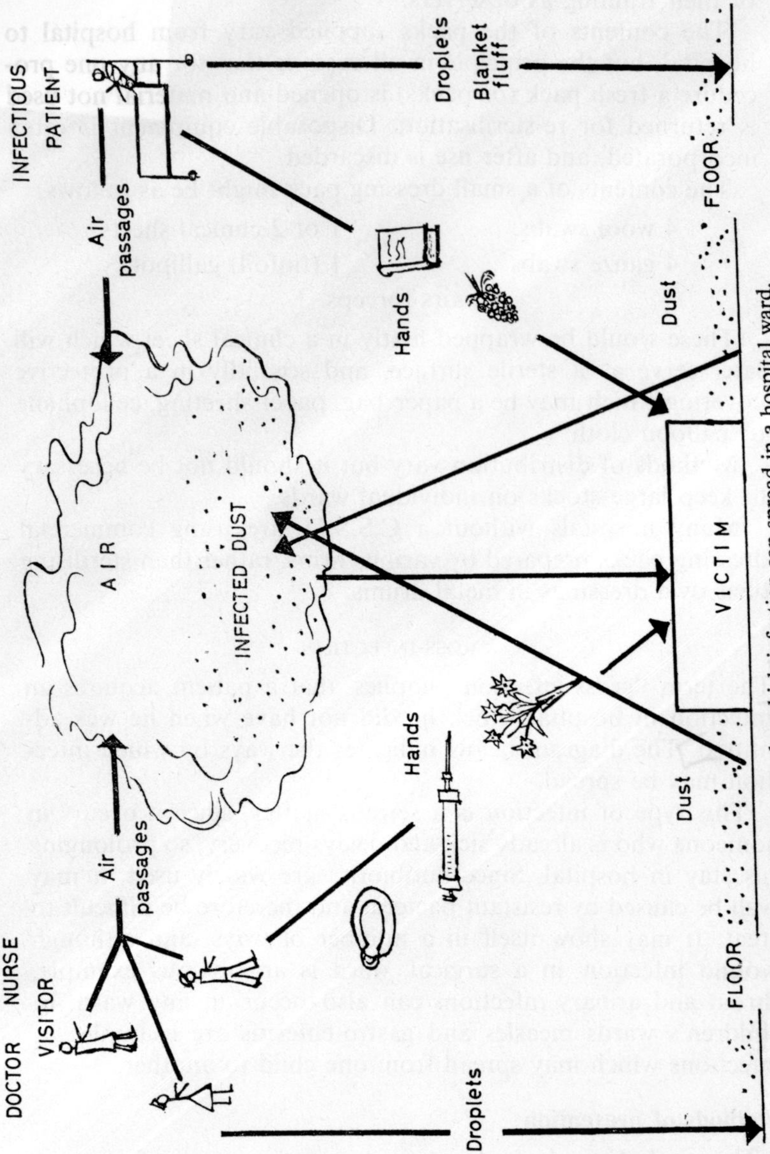

Fig. 23.—The routes by which infection can spread in a hospital ward.

also important and overcrowding must be avoided vision of single rooms or cubicles is a great help for patients when infection has occurred. Adequate ven essential. The use of "dressing" rooms where air can tioned is increasing.

Ward cleaning.—All wards are swept and furniture dusted at least once a day. It is important that this is carried out in such a way that dust is collected and removed, and not merely disturbed and allowed to settle elsewhere. The best method is to use damp or impregnated dusters and vacuum-type sweepers, as hospital dust invariably contains bacteria, some of them pathogenic. Ward floors can be treated with a special oil (spindle oil), but this is only suitable for wood.

Ward staff.—The health of all members of the ward team is important. It is becoming increasingly common for nurses about to work in theatre or in a surgical ward to have nose and throat swabs taken to ensure that they are not harbouring organisms (especially staphylococcus aureus) likely to cause cross-infection. All coughs, colds, septic foci or gastro-intestinal upsets must be reported at once.

Ward routine.—1. Bedmaking: any patient with an infection will contaminate his bedclothes. It is essential that bedmaking should be carried out with care, avoiding excessive shaking of blankets. It is also important that no articles should be transferred from one bed to another or be placed on the floor.

2. Dressings: as any activity in the ward increases the number of bacteria present in the air, it is necessary to restrict this to a minimum for 15 minutes before dressings are done; this applies particularly to cleaning and bedmaking. Dressings are carried out with full aseptic technique (see Chapter XI).

Aseptic technique.—During her training the student nurse will learn many procedures, some of which are carried out with clean equipment—for example, cleaning a patient's mouth—others requiring sterile equipment and an aseptic technique. The latter are necessary when carrying out any dressing on an area where the skin is broken, and for investigations and treatments when it is important that no organisms are introduced—e.g. injections, catheterisation and lumbar puncture.

Certain principles apply for all procedures requiring aseptic technique:

1. All equipment must be sterile.
2. The nurse and doctor should wash and dry their hands.
3. All equipment is handled with forceps (non-touch technique) except when sterile rubber gloves are worn.
4. All dirty dressings must be placed in a suitable closed container as soon as they are removed, and later burnt.
5. The tray or trolley must be cleared, cleaned and re-set with further sterile equipment before proceeding to another patient.

Chapter VIII

MEDICINES AND DRUGS

Substances can be given to the patient to produce a change in his condition; these are loosely termed drugs or medicines. In practice, the term drug is usually reserved for those substances which cannot be obtained without a prescription, and the term medicines for simple substances such as those which may be found in the home. In fact the two terms are synonymous.

All drugs have an official name, but many are marketed by several firms under different proprietary names; throughout this chapter the official name is given first with other names in brackets. Many drugs are controlled by Acts of Parliament; for example:

1. The Dangerous Drugs Act names those which are drugs of addiction. These include:

Opium and its derivatives, e.g. morphine, Papaveretum (Omnopon).
Pethidine hydrochloride (Demerol, Meperidine).
Methadone (Physeptone, Amidone).
Cocaine.
Heroin and Indian Hemp (Diamorphine and Cannabis Indica).

In hospital these drugs are commonly referred to as D.D.A's; by law they may only be given to a patient on a doctor's prescription, which must clearly state the date, the patient's name, the drug, the dose to be given and whether it may be repeated, and which must bear the doctor's signature.

Ward stocks are the responsibility of the sister-in-charge, who orders drugs as needed from the pharmacist; when these are received she must sign for them and store them in a special locked cupboard; the keys must be kept by the sister or acting sister. When drugs are used, accurate records must be maintained and these can be inspected by the pharmacist at any time. Although not required by law, it is normal hospital practice for two nurses to check and administer all dangerous drugs, and in many hospitals one of these must be a State Registered Nurse.

2. Other drugs are mentioned in numbered Schedules of the Poisons Acts; those which apply to medical practice are 1 and 4. Under these Schedules are named drugs which are dangerous if taken in excess. This is a very large group, and includes:

| the barbiturates; | digitalis. |
| the sulphonamides; | codeine |

These drugs must also be prescribed by a doctor in the same way as those controlled by the Dangerous Drugs Act and are ordered from the pharmacy and stored in a locked cupboard inside which is usually the dangerous drug cupboard. Records are often kept, the details varying from one hospital to another; some system of checking should be practised.

3. Many new substances, including the antibiotics, are listed in the Therapeutic Substances Act. These are only available on prescription.

WARD MEDICINES

Drugs not included in either the Dangerous Drugs Act, the Schedules or the Therapeutic Substances Acts are ordered for patients; these are usually stored in a separate cupboard—the medicine cupboard. In hospital they will be prescribed on the patients' treatment sheets and will only be given if so prescribed, although many are available to the general public without a prescription at a chemists or stores; these include tonics, cough mixtures and vitamins. Medicine rounds are carried out several times a day, the medicines being issued according to the treatment sheet.

For details of the specific drugs in use in her ward, the nurse should refer to a pharmacology textbook; the following is simply a guide to some types of drugs which are commonly used.

CLASSIFICATION OF DRUGS IN COMMON USE

1. **Drugs which act on the digestive system.**—Many drugs are available which in some way affect the activities of the digestive system—digestion, absorption and excretion.

(*a*) It is sometimes necessary to give the patient substances normally produced by his own cells, e.g. hydrochloric acid. Alternatively, overactivity may have to be checked, as when the stomach produces too much acid, and an *antacid* is given, e.g. aluminium hydroxide (Aludrox).

(*b*) In constipation, *laxatives* are given to produce evacuation of the bowel contents (see Chapter IX).

When diarrhoea occurs, certain substances are used to control it, e.g. chalk and opium mixture.

(*c*) When vomiting cannot be controlled by simple nursing measures, *anti-emetic* drugs may be used; these include chlorpromazine (Largactil), and many of the anti-histamines. Occasionally it is necessary to make the patient vomit—for example, in some cases of poisoning, and here an *emetic* is given; the simplest is a strong salt-and-water solution.

(*d*) *Carminatives* are substances given to a patient who has discomfort due to swallowing excess air, in an attempt to "bring it up". Peppermint water is a popular remedy.

(*e*) Intestinal worms are treated by various drugs—the *anthelmintics*: theseinclude piperazine (Antepar, Entacyl).

2. **Drugs acting on the nervous system.**—In general these drugs either depress or stimulate the activities of the nervous system.

(*a*) *Depressants* may be divided into those which produce drowsiness or sleep, and those which relieve pain and induce sleep, i.e. the *hypnotics* and *narcotics*. Examples of the former are the barbiturates, e.g. butobarbitone (Soneryl), phenobarbitone (Luminal) and chloral hydrate; and of the latter, morphine.

Drugs which simply relieve pain are called *analgesics*, and a common one is pethidine hydrochloride (Demerol).

Mild analgesics include codeine compound (Veganin) and acetyl salicylic acid (aspirin).

(*b*) *Stimulants* of the nervous system include the amphetamines which have received much publicity as "pep pills". Examples are amphetamine (Benzedrine) and dex-amphetamine (Dexedrine).

Common stimulants freely available to everyone are strong tea and coffee.

(*c*) Drugs acting on the heat-regulating centre are called *anti-pyretics*, common examples being acetyl salicylic acid (aspirin) and sodium salicylate.

115

(d) *Tranquillisers* have a calming effect on the emotions, without necessarily making the patient sleepy. They are commonly used in the treatment of mental illness, and include chlorpromazine (Largactil).

(e) Many drugs act on the autonomic nervous system; one of the commonest is atropine, which may be used for its *anti-spasmodic* and *anti-secretory* effect.

(f) Alcohol acts as a carminative in the stomach and as a depressant to the central nervous system.

3. **Drugs acting on the circulatory system.**—(a) Digitalis. This drug is widely used in many heart conditions, particularly when the rhythm is affected. A common preparation is digoxin (Lanoxin).

(b) Certain drugs act on the vessels and by increasing or decreasing their size, affect the flow of blood to a part; these are called *vasodilators*, e.g. glyceryl trinitrate and *vasoconstrictors*, e.g. adrenalin.

(c) Blood pressure has already been discussed; if it is very high or very low, substances may be given in an attempt to bring it nearer normal. In the former, *hypotensives* are given, e.g. bethanidine sulphate (Esbatal), pentolinium tartrate (Ansolysen) and methyldopa (Aldomet), and in the latter, drugs to raise the blood pressure, e.g. noradrenaline (Levophed).

(d) *Anticoagulants* are used to prevent clot formation within the vessels. One of the best known is heparin, another is warfarin (Marevan).

4. **Drugs acting on the urinary system.**—(a) The normal reaction of urine is slightly acid; it may be necessary to give drugs to alter the reaction. A common mixture is potassium citrate, which makes the urine alkaline.

(b) If water is retained in the body, a *diuretic* is used to increase the urinary output. One group of diuretics concontain mercury, e.g. mersalyl, and a second group are non-mercurial, e.g. frusemide (Lasix).

5. **Drugs acting on the respiratory system.**—(a) *Expectorants* are given to help the patient cough up sputum; numerous substances are used, many common mixtures containing

ipecacuanha. At times an irritating cough may prevent the patient from resting, and in this case a *linctus* is used to depress the cough, e.g. linctus codeine.

(*b*) To relieve spasm of the bronchioles, a *bronchodilator* is ordered, e.g. aminophylline.

(*c*) Substances which stimulate the respiratory centre are a mixture of oxygen and carbon dioxide (inhaled), and many drugs including nikethamide (Coramine).

6. **Hormones.**—These are produced by the endocrine glands and control many body activities. In certain conditions, extracts or synthetic preparations may be given to the patient to increase the amount available.

Examples are insulin, cortisone, adreno-cortico-trophic-hormone (A.C.T.H.) and thyroid extract.

7. **Chemotherapeutics** and **antibiotics** are substances used to control infection. Many have been developed over the last 30 years and include in the first case the sulphonamides, and in the second case the penicillins, the tetracyclines (Aureomycin, Terramycin), streptomycin and others.

8. **Anti-histamines.**—Histamine is normally present in the body in an inert form; following injury, irritation or allergy, this becomes active and can cause abnormal reactions. Should this happen, any one of a large group of drugs—the *anti-histamines* —may be given. Examples are promethazine (Phenergan), mepyramine maleate (Anthisan) and chlorcyclazine hydrochloride (Histantin).

These drugs were originally included in the Schedule lists but have now been transferred to the Part 1, Poisons List. This means that they can be bought without a prescription, but the manufacturers must mark the container "These preparations may cause drowsiness".

9. **Cytotoxic drugs.**—These are used in certain malignant conditions and act by interfereing with cell division. Examples are thio-tepa, 6-mercaptopurine and Busulphan (Myleran).

It is important to remember that many drugs affect more than one system, and that some have unpleasant side-effects.

METHODS OF ADMINISTRATION

The most common way for drugs to be given is in a mixture or tablet which is taken by mouth and swallowed. For various reasons other routes may have to be used; for instance, drugs may be given:

1. By injection: hypodermic;
   intramuscular;
   intravenous;
   intrathecal.
2. Per rectum.
3. By inhalation.
4. As a local application.

Oral administration

Many simple medicines are given by mouth, commonly during the ward medicine round. These are usually taken round on a trolley and in addition to the medicines and tablets she will need, the nurse collects medicine glasses suitable for the doses to be given, and other equipment, including a jug of cold water in case any patient has none by his bed.

The medicines are issued according to the prescription sheets; some medicine bottles need to be shaken before removing the cork, to mix the contents; it is a wise precaution to hold the bottle with the label against the palm of the hand while pouring; this ensures that any drips do not obliterate the label. When measuring the dose, the glass should be held at eye level, as the level of liquid seen through glass is deceptive if looked at from above. The nurse checks the name of the patient and the label on the bottle, pours out the required dose, re-corks the bottle and, after re-checking with the prescription sheet, takes the glass to the patient on a small tray. Tablets are shaken into a disposable container or on to a spoon and checked as above before being given to the patient; if any difficulty in swallowing is experienced, many tablets may be crushed and taken as a powder or dissolved in water. If a medicine has an unpleasant taste or is likely to stain the teeth, it is customary to offer the patient a straw; oily mixtures may be given with a little concentrated fruit juice. The nurse should stay with the patient until he has taken the medicine, and offer him a drink of water or fruit juice if desired.

Glasses and spoons are placed in a bowl of hot soapy water after use—usually on the bottom of the trolley—and rinsed and dried as necessary.

Should any patient refuse a medicine, this must be reported to the ward sister. Children need a firm but kindly approach, and small bribes in the form of a favourite sweet afterwards are preferable to false promises about the taste of the medicine!

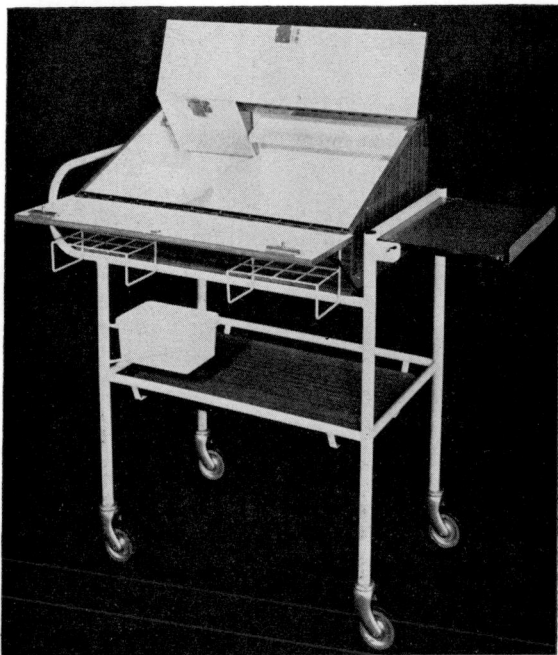

FIG. 24.—Movable Medicine Trolley.
(*Hospital Metalcraft Ltd.*)

During the medicine round, the trolley must be in the nurse's view at all times; should she be called away, it must be removed to a safe place.

At the end of the round, the nurse should wipe all the bottles, place empty ones to one side to be sent to the pharmacy, and if any labels appear indistinct or discoloured, these bottles should also be sent for re-labelling.

A modern piece of equipment is the "movable" medicine cupboard, which serves as a trolley, but can be locked in place when not in use.

When a drug included in the Poisons or Dangerous Drugs Act is to be given by mouth, the rules previously mentioned under these headings must be observed.

When medicines are prescribed, the doctor may use official abbreviations to indicate when or how often a drug is to be given. A few of the more common are given below; it will be noted that the abbreviations are of the Latin wording rather than the English.

Abbreviation	Latin phrase	Meaning
a.c.	ante cibum	Before food
p.c.	post cibum	After food
b.d. (b.i.d.)	bis in die	Twice daily
t.d.s.	ter die summendum	3 times daily
q.i.d. (q.d.s.)	quater in die	4 times daily
q.q.h.	quaquae quater hora	Every 4 hours
—	mane	In the morning
—	nocte	At night
p.r.n.	pro re nata	When necessary
stat.	statim	At once

Injections

Drugs are given by injection for the following reasons:

1. Speed of absorption: drugs given by injection reach the blood stream more quickly than when given by mouth, and are therefore effective more rapidly. Obviously if given intravenously (I.V.)—that is, into the blood stream—the effect is almost instantaneous.

2. Some drugs are inactivated by the acid medium in the stomach, the best example being the earlier penicillins.

3. In cases of persistent vomiting, or when oral administration is contraindicated—for example, after some operations on the stomach.

A. Hypodermic (subcutaneous) injections.—The word hypodermic means under the skin—that is, the drug is given into the subcutaneous tissues; in some areas, e.g. the upper arm, this layer is fairly thick and therefore provides a convenient site. This route is suitable for small amounts of fluid, usually not more than 1 ml. and so only a small syringe is needed; the size of the needle should be 16 to 20.

In most hospitals a central syringe service exists, or sterile disposable syringes are used. If a pre-sterilised syringe is not available, all equipment must be boiled for 5 minutes.

(i) *Preparing the injection.*—The drug is collected and checked with the prescription sheet; it will commonly be dispensed in a single-dose container—i.e. a glass ampoule, in the dose required. Should only a part of the dose supplied be needed, a calculation can be made as follows:

Morphine 15 mg. supplied in 1 ml.
Morphine 10 mg. required.

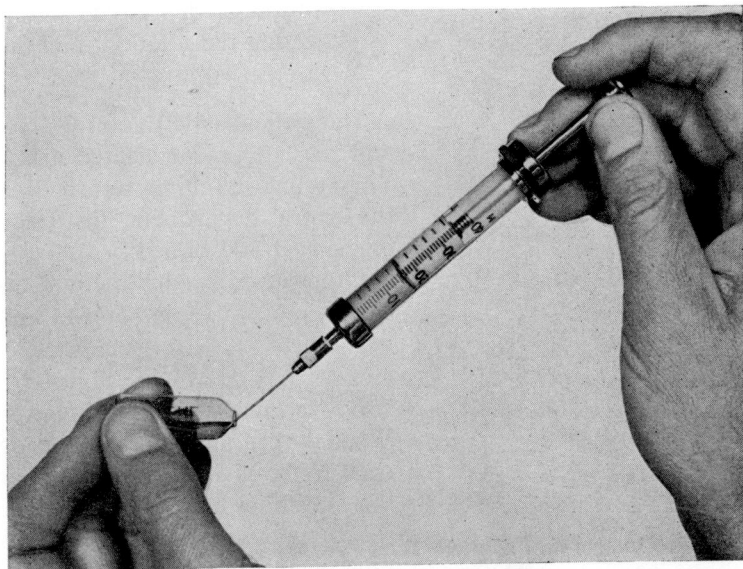

FIG. 25.—Drawing up fluid from a single-dose container.

10 mg. = $\frac{2}{3}$ of 15 mg.
Therefore dose required is $\frac{2}{3}$ ml.

Some drugs given by hypodermic injection are listed in the Dangerous Drugs or Poisons Act, and if so the rules applying to these should be observed. The nurse should wash and dry her hands, open the container with a file and draw up the drug into the syringe.

It is important that the needle does not touch the outside of the container, or any other unsterile object; if this does happen, a new needle must be obtained. The syringe is placed in a sterile receiver, with the needle resting on a dry sterile wool swab.

(ii) *Giving the injection.*—The receiver is taken to the bedside and the prescription sheet re-checked. The procedure is explained to the patient, the area cleansed using a swab dipped in a suitable lotion—e.g., methylated spirit—or an aerosol spray, and air expelled from the syringe. The injection is given by inserting the needle for a short distance under the skin, at an angle of about 40°. The piston is depressed, so injecting the solution, and the needle withdrawn.

The patient is left comfortable, and the equipment cleared away. The syringe is either returned to the central department, discarded or cleaned and boiled.

Drugs given by this method include morphine, atropine and insulin.

B. Intramuscular injections.—When larger amounts of a drug need to be given by injection, or the substance is irritating to the subcutaneous tissues, the intramuscular route is used. Absorption is quicker than by hypodermic injection. The areas used are:

(*a*) The upper arm.

(*b*) The outer aspect of the thigh.

(*c*) The upper outer quadrant of the buttock.

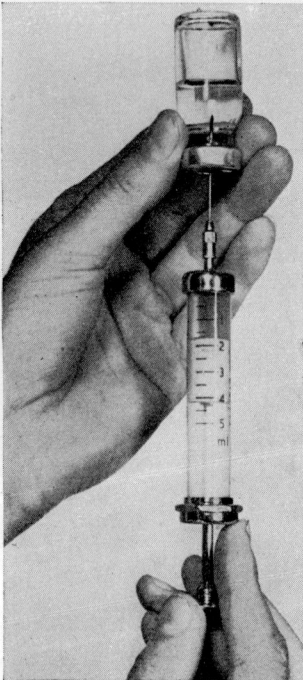
FIG. 26.—Drawing up fluid from a multi-dose container.

A 2 to 5 ml. syringe is used and the needle should be size 1 or 12.

(i) *The preparation* and checking are as described earlier, but sometimes the drug is dispensed in a multi-dose container; in this case the rubber cap is thoroughly cleansed with antiseptic solution and then dried, before being pierced by the needle.

Rubber gloves should be worn by the nurse when handling any solution to which it is possible to develop an allergic reaction, e.g. penicillin, streptomycin and chlorpromazine (Largactil).

(ii) *Giving the injection.*—The procedure is explained to the patient, and if necessary the bed screened. The skin is cleaned and the needle inserted, for about $\frac{3}{4}$ of its length, at right angles to the skin. The piston is withdrawn slightly to make sure the needle is not in a vessel and provided no blood is seen, the injection is given. The needle is then withdrawn and the patient made comfortable; the equipment is then cleared away.

C. **Intravenous injections.**—These are always given by a doctor; the nurse's responsibilities are to collect the necessary equipment for cleaning the skin and giving the injection, to prepare the patient and to assist the doctor if necessary. The size of the syringe and needle will vary according to the amount to be given —this may be as much as 20 mls. The vein chosen is normally in the arm and the nurse may be asked to compress the vessel above the site chosen, to stop the flow of blood in the vein, so making it more prominent. Common drugs given by this route are sodium thiopentone (Pentothal) and heparin. When the injection has been given and the needle withdrawn, firm pressure over the area will stop bleeding.

D. **Intrathecal injections.**—Intrathecal injections are given into the theca, or sub-arachnoid space. Since this involves a lumbar puncture, it will be discussed later (Chapter X). Substances given by this route are antibiotics, anaesthetics or contrast media.

Rectal administration

Not many substances are absorbed satisfactorily by the rectal mucosa, and so this route is not often used. A few drugs are dispensed in suppository form. e.g. aminophylline, and occasionally Pentothal is given rectally before an operation. The amount depends on the patient's weight and age.

Further details of rectal treatments are given in the next chapter.

Drugs given by inhalation

Few substances are given by this method; however, obvious examples are the anaesthetic gases, such as ether, cyclopropane and nitrous oxide, which act on the central nervous system; and amyl nitrite, which is a volatile liquid, and is dispensed in a container which can easily be crushed to release the vapour; it is used in angina pectoris.

Local applications

Many drugs are dispensed for local application, and are available as drops, ointments and lotions.

Drops (guttae) may be prescribed in the treatment of disorders of the eye, the ear and the nose. Common examples are:

(a) For the eye: the antibiotics, and drugs such as sulpha-cetamide (Albucid) and atropine.

(b) For the ear: oily substances to soften wax.

(c) For the nose: ephedrine, which lessens congestion.

Ointments (unguenta).—One way of prescribing a drug for external use is to mix it with a fatty substance to form a semi-solid; many are used in the treatment of skin conditions, especially when the skin is very dry. Eye ointments are also available.

Lotions.—These are watery mixtures for external use, such as calamine lotion and lead lotion (lotio plumbi).

In conclusion, the nurse will have realised that a specific drug may be dispensed in many forms. In fact the crude substance is usually unsuitable in its natural state; for example, digitalis is obtained from the leaf of the foxglove. Drugs are therefore prepared in a way, and in a strength which will make them suitable for administration. Some have already been mentioned, e.g. mixtures, tablets, suppositories, drops and ointments.

Other common preparations are:

Capsules—these are gelatine containers inside which is the drug in powder form; drugs with an unpleasant taste may be dispensed in this way, e.g. many of the barbiturates.

Emulsions—such as liquid paraffin emulsion.

WEIGHTS AND MEASURES

It is becoming increasingly common for drugs to be prescribed in grammes and milligrammes, and liquids measured in litres and millilitres; that is, using the Metric system.

Weight

1000 microgrammes = 1 milligramme
1000 milligrammes = 1 gramme
1000 grammes = 1 kilogramme

From this the nurse will see that it is possible to express doses in the following way:

1 G. (gramme) = 1000 milligrammes
½ G. = 500 milligrammes = 0·5 G.
¼ G. = 250 milligrammes = 0·25 G.

Volume

1000 millilitres (cubic centimetres) = 1 litre

An older system of weights and measures has been used in this country for a long time but is now being replaced by the metric system.

The unit of *weight* is the grain.

Volume

60 minims = 1 drachm
8 drachms = 1 fluid ounce
20 fluid ounces = 1 pint

In hospitals where both systems are in use it may be necessary to convert weights and measures from one system to the other. The following is a guide to the *approximate* values:

125

Weight

10 milligrammes = $\frac{1}{6}$ grain
15 milligrammes = $\frac{1}{4}$ grain
60 milligrammes = 1 grain
1 gramme = 15 grains
1 kilogramme = 2·2 lb.

Volume

1 millilitre = 15 minims
30 millilitres = 1 fluid ounce
600 millilitres = 1 pint
1 litre = $1\frac{3}{4}$ pints (35 fluid ounces)

Chapter IX

SPECIAL CARE OF THE SICK

AIDS TO BREATHING

Administration of oxygen

In health the individual is able to obtain the oxygen he needs from the atmospheric air; in certain conditions it may be necessary to increase the amount available from the normal 20% to about 50% to 60% and in fact 100% oxygen is now in use for patients with severe heart disease. Other conditions include diseases of the respiratory and circulatory systems.

Oxygen is a tasteless, odourless, colourless gas which is supplied compressed in large cylinders. These cylinders may be kept in an oxygen store and the oxygen supplied to the wards by a system of pipes; alternatively, the cylinders themselves may be taken to the wards as needed.

Oxygen is not inflammable, but it readily supports combustion; this means that the nurse's responsibilities include making sure that matches, lighters or anything likely to cause a spark must be removed when oxygen is in use. It is advisable to explain this point to the patients on either side of someone receiving oxygen, and also to his visitors.

As mentioned earlier, carbon dioxide is a stimulant of the respiratory centre and is sometimes given mixed with oxygen (carbon dioxide 5%, oxygen 95%) for short periods, to increase the depth of respiration.

All cylinders are marked with the name of the gas inside and are also distinguishable by the colour—these colours being agreed internationally. For example, oxygen cylinders are black with a white top, while the anaesthetic gases are contained in coloured cylinders.

Before the cylinder can be used, a metal fitting must be screwed into the top; this is normally done by the porter who brings the cylinder to the ward. Attached to this fitting are two gauges—one shows the amount of oxygen in the cylinder, and the other the rate of flow. To open the cylinder a "key" is used; this is kept on the stand and opens the main valve, while the

127

rate of flow is regulated by turning the knob controlling the fine adjustment valve. Oxygen may be required in an emergency and it is therefore very important that every nurse is familiar with the controls.

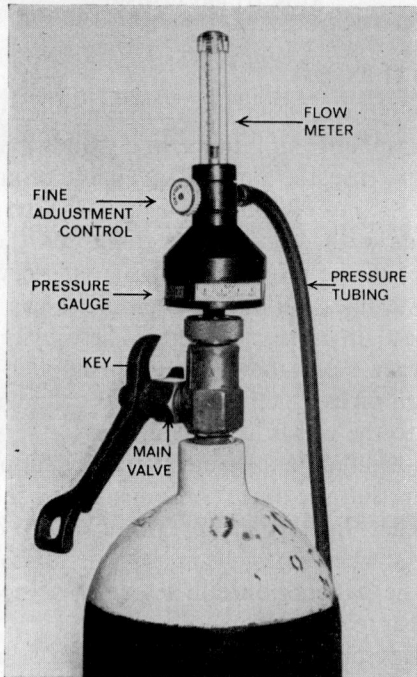

FIG. 27.—Gauges and controls on an oxygen cylinder.

Methods of administration

1. **Disposable polythene masks.**—These are lightweight plastic masks which fit over the patient's nose and mouth. Before placing a mask in position, it is connected to the cylinder using pressure tubing, and the oxygen turned on; the rate of flow for an adult patient is 4 to 6 litres per minute unless otherwise ordered.

If it is the first time the patient has received oxygen, the procedure must be explained carefully, as breathless patients may be further disturbed at the thought of a mask covering the nose and mouth. When it is in position the nurse must check that the tubing is not kinked and that it is not pulling on the mask. The length of time it is left in place will depend entirely on the patient's condition. The amount of oxygen in the cylinder, as registered on the gauge, must be observed at regular intervals and a new cylinder ordered when the gauge shows $\frac{1}{4}$ full. By this method the concentration of oxygen available can be raised from 20% to 45% or 50%. The Ventimask is calibrated to give 27/28% of oxygen.

The mask is used for 1 patient only and is discarded when the patient goes home or is no longer likely to need oxygen.

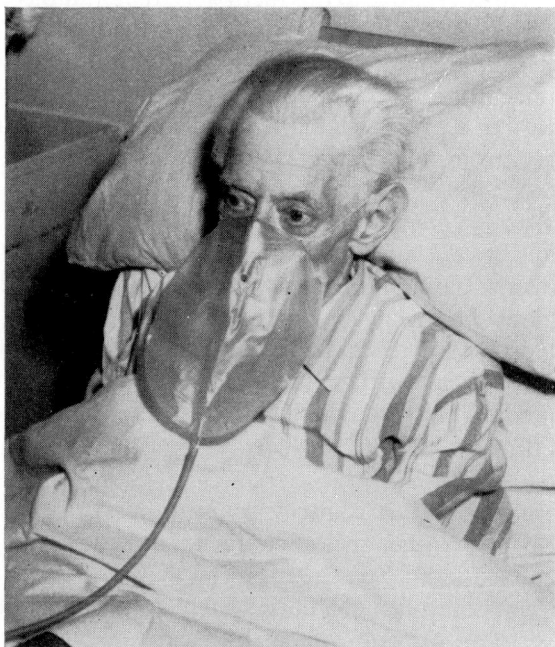

FIG. 28.—Polymask (*The British Oxygen Co. Ltd.*)

2. B.L.B. masks (Boothby, Lovelace and Bulbulian).—These masks are made of rubber and cover either:

(*a*) the nose and mouth, or
(*b*) the nose.

They are not disposable, but apart from this they are used in the same way as the Polymask. After use they must be washed thoroughly in soap and water and may be disinfected.

3. **Nasal catheters.**—Fine catheters may be connected to the oxygen cylinder, using pressure tubing and a Y-shaped connection. Having made sure that the patient's nose is clean and unobstructed, the nurse turns on the oxygen and the catheters are passed along the floor of the nose to the nasopharynx. Occasionally an anaesthetic ointment is used to lubricate the catheters, so facilitating their introduction; alternatively, the lubricant may be white petroleum jelly.

This method is used when a mask cannot be tolerated; one of its advantages is that the patient is able to eat, drink and talk normally. An alternative to this method is to mount pieces of fine rubber tubing on a wire spectacle frame—the Tudor Edward's spectacles. These can now be obtained in a disposable form.

The concentration of available oxygen can be as high as that achieved using a polythene mask; but if the catheters or tubing are merely projecting a short way into the nostrils, it will be much lower.

Humidity.—When air is breathed in, it is moistened, warmed and filtered by the mucous membrane lining the nose. Oxygen under pressure has a drying effect on the membrane, and for this reason many physicians prefer oxygen to be passed through tepid water before reaching the patient. This is achieved by means of a special bottle containing water which is often part of the standard oxygen equipment; this fitting may also incorporate a flow meter.

4. **Oxygen tent.**—If it is necessary to administer oxygen for long periods, or other methods are not tolerated, the patient may be nursed in an oxygen tent.

These tents are plastic canopies fitted to a metal frame and connected to an oxygen cylinder by means of pressure tubing. The canopies are made so that it is possible to tuck the edges well under the mattress; openings are provided through which the nurse can give attention to the patient—these openings are usually secured by zips. Since the temperature will rise rapidly, due to loss of body heat in a confined space, some cooling mechanism is provided; this may be an electrically controlled unit, or the oxygen may be passed through a tank containing ice before reaching the tent. The temperature should not rise above 20° C. (68° F.).

130

The oxygen is turned on and the flow adjusted before the canopy is placed in position; the rate is then maintained at approximately 10 litres per minute for about 10 minutes, to "flush" the tent with oxygen; at the end of this time the flow is reduced to 6 to 8 litres per minute. If at any time the canopy is removed—for instance when the patient is washed—the tent must be "flushed" again when re-erected.

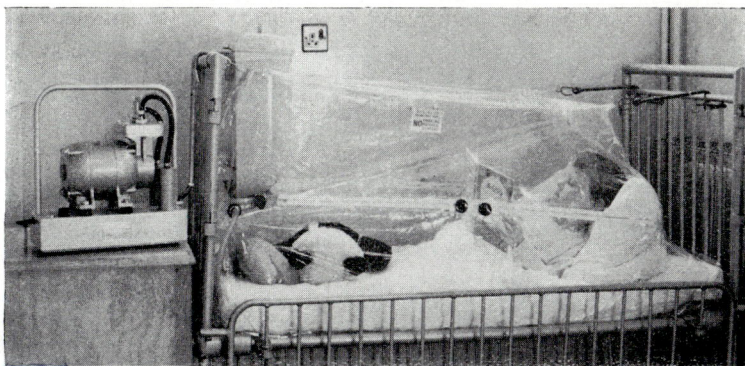

Fig. 29.—Humidaire Junior Oxygen Tent (*Vickers Ltd.*).

The nurse's responsibilities include careful observation of the patient's condition, the amount of oxygen in the cylinder and the rate of flow; she must also re-fill the ice-box when necessary, and empty the drip tray.

The concentration of oxygen available in an oxygen tent may be as high as 60%.

Occasionally an atomiser may be incorporated in the tubing, so that a fine spray of water is added to the atmosphere in the tent; antibiotics or detergent substances may be prescribed and administered in the atomiser. This is most commonly seen in a children's ward.

Inhalations

For those patients who have difficulty in breathing, due to congestion of the upper respiratory tract, steam may be used to loosen the secretions and relieve congestion. Certain substances, which vaporise, may be added to very hot water to assist this process. These include Tincture of Benzoin Compound (Friars Balsam), 3·5 mls. to 600 mls. of water, and Menthol, 2 to 3 crystals to 600 mls. of water.

In many cases it is necessary to provide the patient with a sputum carton and paper handkerchiefs.

1. **Steam inhalation.**—(*a*) In hospital a special container is used —Nelson's inhaler. The patient is made comfortable and supported in the sitting position, the procedure being explained to him.

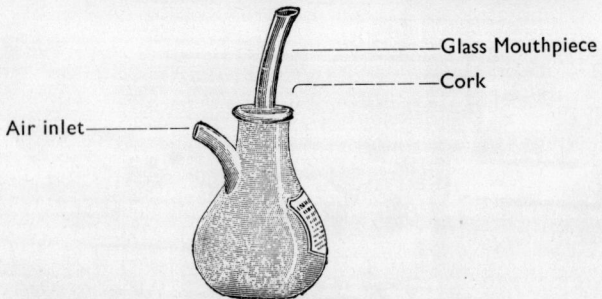

Glass Mouthpiece

Cork

Air inlet

FIG. 30.—Nelson's Inhaler (*Allen & Hanburys Ltd.*)

The inhaler is filled with boiling water to the level of the air inlet, placed in a cover and stood in a bowl with a flat base; the glass mouthpiece is covered with gauze to prevent the patient's lips being burnt. The drug, if prescribed, is measured and is added to the water on reaching the patient's bedside—the reason for this is that the substances used are volatile and are given off very quickly. The cork and mouthpiece are replaced, making sure that the latter is pointing in the opposite direction from the air inlet. The patient is instructed to place his lips around the mouthpiece and breathe in through his mouth and out through his nose. The inhalation will be effective for 7 to 10 minutes and may be repeated every 4 hours.

This type of inhalation is not suitable for the very young, the elderly or mentally confused or very ill patients.

After use the inhaler is emptied and the mouthpiece sterilised. The stains from tincture of benzoin compound can easily be removed using methylated spirit.

(*b*) When steam is used to lessen congestion in the nose or sinuses, or if a Nelson's inhaler is not available, it is possible to carry out this form of treatment using an ordinary large jug. The preparation of the patient and the inhalation are the same as before, except that it is advisable to place a folded towel around the jug, so forming a funnel, and if applicable to tell the patient to breathe in through his nose.

2. **Steam tent.**—Some patients need increased humidity for a longer period of time than can be provided by a steam inhalation. For these patients it is possible to erect a steam tent by arranging sheets around a frame so that a canopy is formed over the head of the bed. Steam is introduced by means of a large electric kettle situated outside, with a long spout which projects into the tent; it is important that the spout is placed so that steam is not being projected directly towards the patient. A thermometer is hung inside and the temperature maintained at 21° C. (70° F.). The top pillow must be protected by placing a waterproof pillow case under the cotton case, and the patient is usually nursed in the sitting position. The nurse must see that a bed table is placed in front of him for essential items as he will be unable to reach his locker.

The nurse's responsibilities include observations of the patient's condition and frequent changing of personal and bed linen when these become damp. She must also refill the kettle with hot water at regular intervals.

3. **Special apparatus.**—It has already been mentioned that steam inhalations are unsuitable for the very young. As an increase in humidity is often required in nursing infants with upper respiratory tract infections, special tents have been designed which are similar to small oxygen tents. Oxygen or air is used, together with an atomiser which can produce humidity of up to 100%. One type is called a Croupette and another is the Humidaire.

Breathing Exercises and Postural Drainage

In health, no problems arise with regard to full expansion of the lungs, but in certain conditions it may be necessary to teach the patient how to breathe properly—i.e. to do breathing exercises—in order to secure adequate ventilation. These conditions

133

include some diseases of the respiratory system, and before and after major surgery. In many hospitals these exercises will be taught by a physiotherapist, but at times the nursing staff may have to assume this responsibility. The exercises are aimed mainly at expanding the lower lobes of the lungs; the patient is asked to breathe deeply, and the amount of expansion can be assessed by placing the hands over the lower ribs and feeling the movements of the chest wall.

When excessive secretions collect in the lower respiratory tract, the patient is helped to expectorate by placing him in a suitable position to drain the affected part by gravity. The position varies, but is often achieved by blocking the foot of the bed, or by asking the patient to lie across his bed with his head and chest hanging over the side. This is called postural drainage. The term "clapping" is used to describe the treatment given by physiotherapists to help loosen the secretions and consists of percussion of the chest wall.

AIDS TO FEEDING

It is possible to do without solid food for several days with few ill effects, but adequate fluids must be given to prevent dehydration and electrolyte imbalance. These fluids may be introduced via the alimentary tract, or if this is not possible, intravenously or subcutaneously. An intake and output chart is usually maintained if the patient is receiving supplementary fluids by any route.

1. **Intra-gastric feeding.**—Whenever possible the intra-gastric route is used and fluids given via a tube—usually a Ryle's tube, which may be rubber or plastic.

This is passed into the oesophagus or stomach, via the nose or mouth, and the equipment needed is not necessarily sterile. The patient is made comfortable and the procedure explained. The tube is lubricated or moistened and gently passed either along the floor of the nose, or to the back of the mouth, and the patient is asked to co-operate by swallowing when he feels the tip of the tube in his throat; if allowed, sips of water will help him. Occasionally the patient may feel nauseated and retch— in this case he should be asked to take deep breaths in through the mouth. The nurse continues to pass the tube for the desired length; some tubes are marked, but a rough guide to the length required to reach the stomach may be obtained by measuring from the bridge of the nose to the lower end of the sternum—approximately 40 cms. in the average adult. The pharynx is common to both the respiratory and digestive systems and so it is possible for the tip of the tube to enter the larynx. In the conscious patient this is marked by a fit of coughing, but in the unconscious patient with a poor cough reflex this may not occur, and the nurse must make sure that the tube is in the stomach before giving fluids. This can be done by attaching a syringe to the end of the tube and testing the aspirate with litmus paper; if the tube is in the stomach, the reaction of the secretion will be acid—that is, blue litmus will turn red.

When the tube is in position, fluids may be given at regular intervals; it is advisable to begin and end the feed with 20 to 30 mls. of water to clear the tube. The feed itself will vary in amount and content, but, commonly, fortified milk is given for its nutritional value. It may be introduced in several ways:

(*a*) by using a large syringe;

(*b*) by attaching a funnel to the open end of the tube and allowing the feed to run in by gravity, or

(*c*) by using suitable apparatus, so that the fluid drips down the tube at a steady rate, e.g. 40 to 60 drops per minute; milk is commonly given this way to patients with peptic ulcers. The apparatus required is shown below.

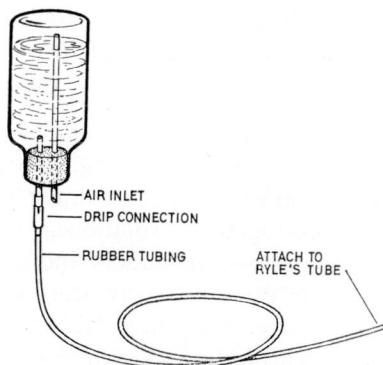

AIR INLET
DRIP CONNECTION
RUBBER TUBING
ATTACH TO RYLE'S TUBE

FIG. 31.—Apparatus for Intra-gastric Feeding.

Between feeds, the end of the tube is closed with a spigot and it will be more comfortable for the patient if the tube is lightly strapped to his cheek.

Patients being fed in this way need frequent attention to their mouths, which will otherwise become very dry.

2. Rectal Infusion.—Few substances are absorbed by the rectal mucosa, but it is possible to give water, saline and some drugs by this route. The preparation of the patient is important as the fluid will not be retained if the rectum is loaded with faeces; if the patient has not had his bowels opened recently, he should be given a suppository or a small enema; he should also be given the opportunity of passing urine before the infusion is started.

The apparatus required is similar to that shown above, but a different type of container may be used, and a catheter, size 6 to 8 (English gauge) replaces the Ryle's tube; this is not a sterile procedure. The fluid given is tap water or saline, which is prepared at body temperature. The nurse explains what she is going to do, the bed is screened and the patient asked to turn on to his left side. The container is filled, hung on the drip stand and fluid allowed to run through the apparatus to expel air; the clip is then closed and the catheter lubricated and passed 7·5–10 cms. into the rectum. The clip is opened to allow the fluid to drip in at a steady rate of not more than 40 drips per minute. If the tubing is strapped lightly to the patient's thigh, he will be able to alter his position as desired without dislodging the catheter; the nurse will have to check from time to time that he is not sitting on the tubing and that the catheter is still in position. The infusion is discontinued when the required amount of fluid has been given, or if it is not being retained.

3. Intravenous infusion.—The method of introducing fluids into a vein is a common one; the substances used must be sterile and include saline and glucose (dextrose) solutions.

The nurse's responsibilities are to prepare the patient and the equipment, to assist the doctor while the infusion is being set up, to see that the patient receives the correct amount of fluid at the prescribed rate, and to discontinue the procedure when necessary.

The procedure is explained to the patient and a bedpan or urinal offered, and any necessary nursing care carried out so that he need be disturbed as little as possible in the early stages of the infusion. Whenever possible the doctor will choose a vein in the lower part of the arm or leg, so that the patient's movements are not restricted too much. If the arm is chosen, it is wise to arrange the patient's gown or pyjama jacket so that the arm is free; this will make his toilet and change of personal linen easier if the infusion is continued over a long period. If the leg is used, the bedclothes are arranged in a suitable way and a small cradle made available.

The equipment necessary includes a suitable cleansing lotion for the skin, sterile swabs, towels and instruments, the fluid to be given, and a "giving set" which is pre-sterilised and is often disposable. Occasionally it is necessary to "cut down" to reach a vein, and in this case suitable instruments should be provided.

It may be necessary to apply a light splint to immobilise the limb, the area round the needle being left uncovered so that observation of the site is possible.

Once the infusion is in progress the nurse must make sure that the patient is comfortable and report any complaints of pain or discomfort; the rate must be maintained as ordered, and if it stops or any swelling is observed around the needle (i.e. fluid running into the tissues and not into the vein) the sister or nurse in charge must be informed. The infusion is more likely to run satisfactorily if the limb is kept warm and in a relaxed, comfortable position.

When the bottle is nearly empty, it must be replaced if the infusion is to be continued; in many hospitals a senior nurse must be present when the new bottle is put up. The type of fluid is as ordered, the infusion is turned off and the apparatus changed from one bottle to the other, care being taken not to contaminate that part of the set which is going inside the new container. It is then restarted at the appropriate rate.

When the infusion is to be discontinued, the nurse turns it off, gently withdraws the needle and applies a sterile dressing to the site. The patient is left comfortable and the apparatus is either discarded or cleaned and returned for re-sterilising. It is important to note and record the exact amount that has been given.

4. Subcutaneous infusion.—A less common method of giving fluids is by subcutaneous infusion; here fluid is run slowly into the subcutaneous tissues and its absorption aided by the addition of a tissue enzyme, hyaluronidase (Hyalase). Since the fluid is absorbed slowly, only small amounts can be given by this route and it is therefore a more common procedure in a children's ward.

The apparatus required is sterile and is similar to that needed for an intravenous infusion—occasionally two needles are inserted at the same time, and in this case a Y-shaped connection and extra rubber tubing are needed.

The patient is made comfortable, an explanation given and the site exposed; the most common site being the outer aspect of the thigh. The nurse who is to put up the infusion washes and dries her hands, assembles the apparatus and runs a little of the fluid (usually saline) through the tubing and needle to expel air. The skin is cleansed and the needle inserted in the same way as for a subcutaneous (hypodermic) injection. The Hyalase may either be added to the contents of the container or be injected into the tubing just above the needle as soon as the infusion is running.

The rate at which the fluid is given is determined by the rate of absorption but is rarely more than 30 drops per minute; no undue swelling should be obvious around the needle, which may be held in place by strapping or sellotape. It is very important that full aseptic technique is maintained as infection can easily be introduced into the tissues. When the infusion is discontinued, the needle is withdrawn and a sterile dressing applied.

Notes on fluids

Normal saline is a 0·9% solution of salt and water; this concentration is the same as that found in blood and tissue fluids. Weaker solutions of saline such as $\frac{1}{2}$ normal strength (0·45%) and $\frac{1}{5}$ normal (0·18%) are commonly combined with dextrose. Hartmann's, Ringer's and Darrow's solutions contain other salts such as potassium and calcium and can be used to correct electrolyte imbalance.

Dextrose solutions are irritating to the subcutaneous tissues and are not given by this route.

AIDS TO BOWEL FUNCTION

People's habits vary. The majority of healthy individuals empty their bowels each day; however, it is equally normal for this to happen twice daily, or once every three days. The colon is stimulated by the intake of food, especially after the first meal of the day; provided the diet is suitable, no artificial stimulation is necessary. The foods likely to increase peristalsis are those containing cellulose (or "roughage"), that is, complex carbohydrates. The producers of one of the popular breakfast cereals make use of this fact in their advertisements. An adequate fluid intake is also necessary—as is exercise.

Defaecation (the passing of faeces) is under voluntary control from about the age of eighteen months, nerve-endings in the rectum being stimulated by the presence of faeces and producing the desire to defaecate. In some seriously ill, or old people, control may be lost, faeces being passed involuntarily as in infants; this is termed faecal incontinence.

The terms constipation and diarrhoea are sometimes mis-used. Constipation means that faeces are harder than usual—due to excess re-absorption of water—causing pain and difficulty on defaecation. It is often due to failure to maintain regular bowel habits; other causes being insufficient fluid, unsuitable diet and, occasionally, disease. Diarrhoea is the reverse—the faeces being almost fluid; because of this the number of bowel actions per day is increased. Causes include unsuitable food, infection and, again, disease.

Patients in hospital may be confined to bed, may be drinking less than usual, and may not be able to eat their normal diet. It follows that there is often some disturbance of normal bowel habits—namely, constipation. A further inhibitory factor is the bedpan; it is uncomfortable, unnatural and even though bed curtains or screens are provided, is very different from the normal privacy of the toilet at home.

A record is kept of the patient's bowel actions and to prevent constipation the following may have to be used:

(*a*) Aperients.
(*b*) Suppositories.
(*c*) Enemas.

Aperients
Aperients fall into four categories:
1. **Lubricants** such as liquid paraffin. These are mild and do not

139

actually increase peristalsis—they merely, as their name suggests, ease the passage of faeces.

2. Bowel irritants such as cascara. These are stronger and initiate forceful peristalsis by direct action on the bowel wall. They take several hours to have effect and because of this are usually given in the late evening.

. **Saline aperients.**—These act by drawing water into the bowel, so increasing the faecal mass and stimulating peristalsis. The commonest is magnesium sulphate (Epsom salts). They act more quickly than the last category and arc given first thing in the morning.

4. "Bulk" laxatives.—These are substances which have no food value, but absorb water during their passage through the body, and so add bulk to the faeces. An example is the proprietary preparation Isogel granules.

When constipation is a problem, the doctor will prescribe a suitable aperient. He will often ask the patient if they are in the habit of taking laxatives and, if so, will prescribe one which suits them. It is inadvisable to give, or take, aperients over a long period of time without medical advice.

Suppositories

These are cone-shaped objects, 2 to 3 cm in length; they are inserted into the rectum, where they dissolve.

The simplest is the glycerine suppository; this consists of a gelatine base, with glycerine added; in the bowel the glycerine acts in the same way as the saline aperients.

A suppository which is frequently used is known by the trade name of Dulcolax. This contains drugs which are bowel irritants, and has a more forceful action than glycerine.

Special suppositories may be used in other conditions, e.g. Anusol—which are used for patients with pain and rectal bleeding due to haemorrhoids.

Insertion of suppositories.—A careful explanation is necessary and the bed curtains are drawn before proceeding. To help the patient to relax he can be instructed to breathe through his mouth; this prevents tightening of the anal sphincter, and so makes the introduction of the suppository easier. The patient is asked to lie on his left side with his knees drawn up; the nurse puts on a rubber glove or finger-stall, and using her index finger gently pushes the suppository into the rectum. Glycerine suppositories are easier to insert if dipped in warm water first—this is not necessary for Dulcolax. After 20 to 30 minutes, the patient will either go to the ward toilet or use a bedpan or commode.

Used finger-stalls are discarded. Rubber gloves are washed in hot soapy water, rinsed and sterilised before being used for another patient.

Disposable gloves are now available.

Enemas

An enema is the introduction of fluid into the rectum. The use of evacuant enemas has now been largely superseded by suppositories; however, the nurse may be asked to given an enema, and must be familiar with the types of fluid used, and with the equipment and technique. Before giving any enema the patient must be given the opportunity to empty his bladder, as this will lessen discomfort.

The most common reason for this procedure is to empty the lower bowel, e.g. before certain operations and investigations. In this case the following may be used:

(*a*) **Disposable enema.**—One type consists of 128 mls. of fluid in a plastic container, with a non-traumatic rectal tube attached. The fluid is distilled water, with sodium diphosphate and sodium phosphate added; this solution acts as a bowel irritant, and produces an evacuation of faeces.

The directions are on the container, and read:

"Remove cap and lubricate tube; insert in rectum; squeeze gently until all fluid is dispelled and discard container."

The pack, as described, is suitable for an adult patient; smaller amounts are given to children.

The lubricant used is usually yellow petroleum jelly, and the position of the patient during the procedure is the same as for the insertion of suppositories, care being taken not to expose the patient unduly. If he is confined to bed, a bedpan and toilet

141

paper should be available; on removing the bedpan, the patient is given a bowl of water to wash his hands, and is made comfortable. The nurse takes the bedpan to the sluice and inspects the contents. She should note the amount of faeces passed and any abnormality. A report is made to sister.

This method has advantages over the traditional methods in that a smaller amount of fluid is used, thereby lessening discomfort, and no elaborate equipment is needed.

(b) **Tap water, and soap and water.**—In these cases, up to 1200 mls. of fluid may be used, at body temperature.

If soap and water is to be given, it is either prepared by adding water to soap solution, or by dissolving a small cube of green soft soap in boiling water, cold water being added to reach the desired temperature and amount.

For a child, the amount of fluid used is 30 mls. per year of age.

The apparatus used is a funnel, a length of rubber tubing, a connection and a rubber catheter, size 8 to 12.

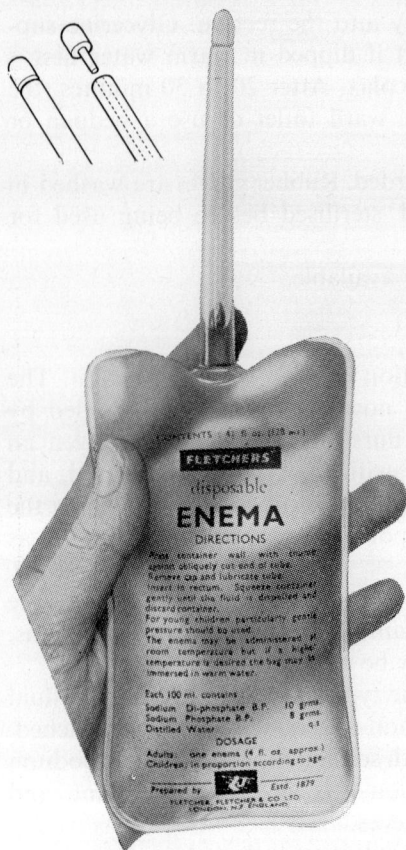

FIG. 32.—Disposable Enema (*Fletcher Fletcher & Co. Ltd.*).

Having collected all her equipment, the nurse screens the bed and explains the procedure to the patient. His position is that already described for other rectal treatments. It is advisable to protect the bed by placing a small towel and waterproof sheeting under the patient's buttocks.

The catheter is lubricated with yellow petroleum jelly; air is expelled from the apparatus by pouring fluid into the funnel until it runs out of the eye of the catheter. The tubing is then compressed either with the fingers or a spring clip, and the catheter gently inserted 7·5–10 cms into the rectum. The tubing is released, and the fluid (water or soap and water), poured into the funnel until the required amount has been given. The funnel is held approximately 30 cms above the level of the mattress.

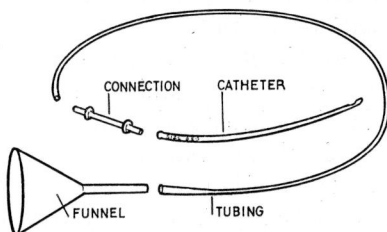

FIG. 33.—Enema Apparatus.

Having given the enema the catheter is withdrawn.

The patient may feel discomfort, but if he complains of pain the nurse should stop immediately, and report to sister, the patient being left in a comfortable position. A bedpan is given as soon as the patient wishes, and the toilet paper placed within reach.

On removing the bedpan, the nurse takes it to the sluice and inspects the contents; she should note the amount of faeces passed, the approximate amount of fluid returned and any abnormalities present. A report is then made to sister.

Following the procedure, the patient is given an opportunity to wash his hands, and is made comfortable. All equipment used is carefully washed and rinsed; the best way to clean the inside of a catheter is to hold it under a running tap, so that the water passes from the "eye" end, down the tube. The catheter, and any other articles contaminated by faeces (e.g. the receiver), are then sterilised by boiling for 5 minutes, alternatively, all equipment is returned to the C.S.S.D.

Other reasons for giving enemas are:

(a) To soften faeces.
(b) To introduce drugs or other substances.
(c) To lessen raised intracranial pressure.
(d) For the relief of "wind" (or flatus).

The method, equipment, position and care of the patient and the observations to be made are similar to those already mentioned. Where there are differences in detail, these will be described.

(*a*) **Olive oil enema.**—This is used to soften faeces in severe constipation, or occasionally as a post-operative measure to prevent pain on defaecation following some gynaecological or rectal operations.

180–240 mls. of warm olive oil is given; this is to be retained for several hours, and so must be given slowly. For this reason a small catheter and a shorter piece of rubber tubing are used. The simplest method of warming the oil is to stand the container in a bowl of hot water, but care must be taken to see that it is not above 38° C. (100° F.) when given.

The oil is followed, 4 to 6 hours later, by a soap and water enema. A disposable arachis oil enema is available.

(*b*) In conditions in which the bowel wall is inflamed, a hydrocortisone or a starch and opium enema may be ordered. These substances act directly on the mucous membrane, and lessen pain and discomfort. As they are to be retained, they should be given slowly.

Hydrocortisone.—120–180 mls. of hydrocortisone solution is given; this acts by lessening the inflammatory process. This is also available in a disposable container.

Starch and opium.—2–4 mls. of tincture of opium is given in 120–180 mls. of starch solution. The starch is similar to the domestic variety, and is prepared in the same way, making sure that the solution is thin enough to run through the catheter.

(*c*) **Magnesium sulphate** given per rectum produces a watery stool; this reduces the amount of circulating fluid and so indirectly relieves raised intracranial pressure. In many hospitals other methods are now in use, e.g. the administration of urea by mouth or intravenously, which produces a diuresis.

If used, 120–180 mls. of 25% magnesium sulphate solution is given. This solution is available in a disposable container (50% in 130 ml.).

(*d*) **Turpentine or ox-bile enema.**—These are rarely used nowadays, but may be given to relieve distension due to flatus. This type of enema is termed "carminative" or "anti-spasmodic".

Turpentine—up to 30 mls. may be given, either thoroughly mixed with 600 mls. of soap and water solution, or with 60–120 mls. of olive oil. Turpentine is an irritant, and the skin around the anus should be protected with petroleum jelly. The nurse can judge the efficacy of this treatment by the patient's own comments, and by feeling his abdomen.

Ox-bile—7–15 mls. is given, usually in a pint of soap and water solution.

Anthelmintic enemas are an old method of treating intestinal worms. The solution used was hypertonic saline.

The use of a flatus tube

This is another method of relieving flatus. There are various sizes of flatus tube, which differ from catheters in that the opening is at the end rather than on the side of the tube.

The tube is lubricated, and inserted up to 20 cms into the rectum and sigmoid colon. If desired, the open end is attached to a funnel, or weighted and placed in a bowl of water. The tube is removed after 10 minutes, and the patient made comfortable. If necessary the procedure is repeated.

Abdominal distension due to flatus is less common today, as patients get up much sooner after operations.

COLOSTOMY AND ILEOSTOMY

One of the operations which is sometimes performed on the alimentary tract is to make an artificial opening for the passage of faeces on to the front of the abdomen. This opening is called a colostomy when the colon is involved, and an ileostomy when the small intestine is opened. These operations are performed when some disease, obstruction or abnormality of the intestine makes normal defaecation difficult or impossible.

Care of colostomy

For the first few days following operation, the area is treated as any surgical wound—that is, with full aseptic technique; this is to assist healing of the skin around the opening. At operation a tube may be inserted into the opening to drain faeces and so avoid contamination of the area while healing is taking place. Within a few days this tube will be removed and the faeces will be discharged on to the skin; it is then necessary to provide some covering to collect the faeces. This may be in the form of unsterile dressings—layers of gauze and wool, covered with a

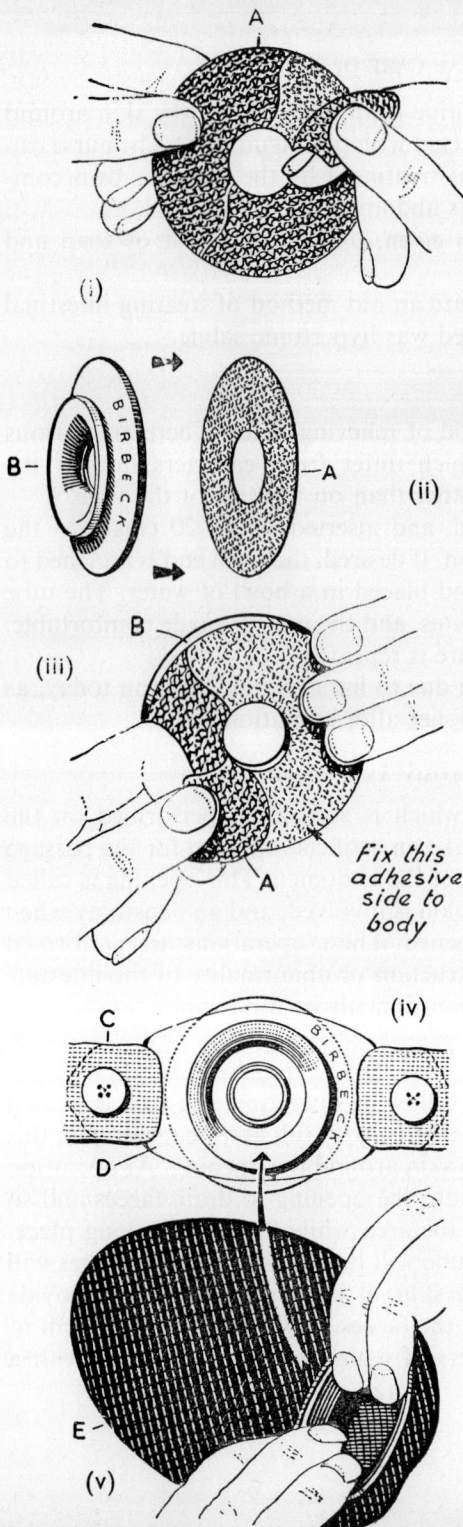

Fig. 34.—Fitting an ileostomy or colostomy appliance.

(i) Remove cloth protection on one side of the adhesive plaster (A) and place the sticky side firmly to the flat side of the rubber face-piece (B). (*See note 2.*)

(ii) Next ensure that the centre hole of the rubber face-piece (B) is the correct size for the bowel opening. The rubber opening can be enlarged by careful cutting round with scissors.

(iii) Remove the second cloth backing from the plaster on the face-piece and place the sticky side thus revealed firmly and comfortably over the bowel opening ensuring adhesion to the body by even pressure. (*See notes* 1 *and* 2).

(iv) Next place plastic retaining shield (D) over the rubber face-piece and secure the waistband (C) round the body. Adjust to a comfortable pressure.

(v) If a rubber bag is to be used, place in position by stretching the bag opening over the lip of the face-piece (B) so that the bag is retained in the face-piece groove.

Fix this adhesive side to body

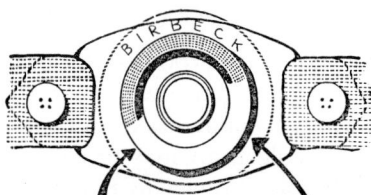

Fig. 34.—(*Continued*).

(vi) and (vii). If the plastic disposable bag (G) is used, slip it through the rubber retaining ring (H) and pull the plastic and the ring over the face-piece groove.

Notes:
1. *Should the skin become sore, a protective coating of Nobecutane spray[1] can be sprayed on the skin round the bowel opening.*
2. *Some patients prefer to use the rubber face-piece without the double-sided plasters, securing it in position with the waistband only.*

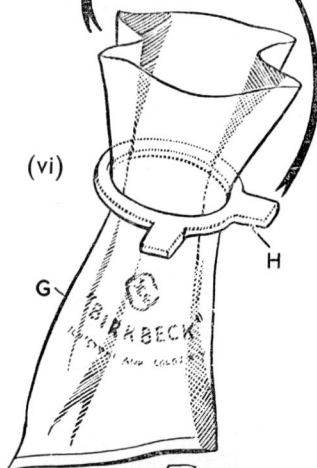

[1]A sterile transparent dressing for surgical use (*Evans Medical Ltd.*).

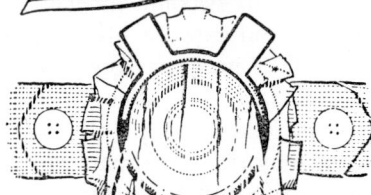

(*Fig. 34 reproduced by courtesy of J. G. Franklin & Sons, Ltd.*)

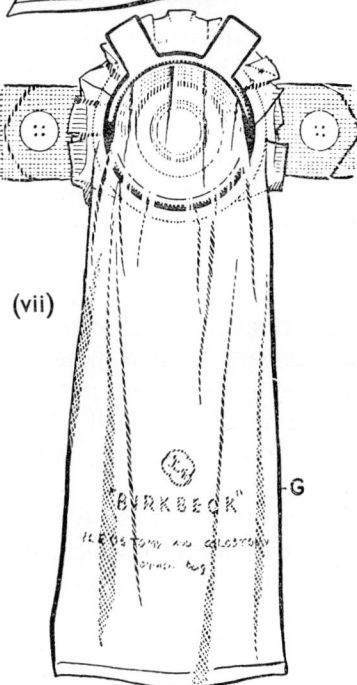

(vi)

(vii)

piece of waterproof material and a bandage, or a plastic bag. At first, the nurse will change the dressings or bag, and clean the skin using moist wool swabs—the gut is insensitive to pain, so the colostomy may be cleaned gently; it may be necessary to apply an ointment to the skin if the area around the opening becomes red. Most of the bags used today are made of a cheap plastic material, and are discarded after use. Many types and sizes are in use, and it is important to choose the right one for each individual patient.

Occasionally this operation is performed as a temporary measure, but sometimes it is permanent and the gut below it may be removed. In either case the idea of an opening for faeces on the abdomen is a great shock for the patient and needs careful explanation beforehand. In the case of a permanent colostomy, many ward sisters feel that a good way of helping the patient to adjust is to arrange a visit from an ex-patient who has managed a colostomy for some time. The patient's reaction to his condition depends to a large extent on the nursing staff and their reactions. One of the nurse's main responsibilities is to help him become independent, so that he knows how to regulate and care for his colostomy in his own home.

It will be necessary both in and out of hospital to adjust the diet so that foods likely to produce loose stools are avoided; these include fruits, highly spiced foods and alcohol.

The majority of patients with a colostomy can lead a perfectly normal life and those around them will rarely know of their condition.

Care of an ileostomy

The principles of care are the same as for colostomy, but the management is often more difficult. This is partly due to the fact that the opening is in the small intestine where the contents are normally more fluid, and also because this operation may be performed in young adults for a chronic inflammatory condition of the colon, and they may find it harder to adjust. A third factor is that the small intestine secretes digestive juices containing enzymes which, when discharged with the faeces, irritate the skin causing reddening and soreness. For this reason it is usual to protect the skin around the opening with an ointment such as aluminium paste.

To make the faeces less fluid, more bulk is given in the diet, usually in the form of cellulose (Isogel).

It cannot be emphasised too strongly that these patients need much reassurance, support and understanding.

Chapter X

AIDS TO DIAGNOSIS AND TREATMENT

Many procedures and tests are carried out in the wards and departments which either help the doctor to make a diagnosis, or form part of the patient's treatment. It is convenient to divide these into three groups:

(1) Those carried out by the nursing staff.
(2) Those performed in the ward by the doctor, but for which the nurse has certain responsibilities.
(3) Those usually carried out away from the ward, which involve the preparation of the patient and his care later.

In all cases, a full explanation must be given to the patient, to put him at ease and to obtain his co-operation. In many cases privacy is essential.

Group 1

CATHETERISATION

A small catheter (about size 6 E.G.) may be passed via the urethra, either to obtain a specimen of urine, or to empty the bladder. The articles used must be sterile, and care is necessary when carrying out this procedure as it is very easy to introduce infection into the urinary tract. If a male patient is to be catheterised, this is usually carried out by a doctor or male nurse. The catheter used is made of either rubber or plastic and if it is to be left in position a self-retaining type is used. This is usually a Foley catheter, the end of which can be inflated to keep it in position.

A good light is essential and as natural lighting is insufficient an Anglepoise lamp or bell lamp is brought to the bedside. The patient is made comfortable, lying on her back; the bedclothes are turned back and a small blanket or bed jacket placed across the patient's chest. She is asked to flex her knees and hips and lie with her legs apart, and waterproof sheeting and a towel are placed under the buttocks. The nurse puts on a mask and washes and dries her hands. Sterile towels or clinical sheets are placed in position over the patient's thighs and a sterile receiver placed between her legs. The vulva is swabbed, using cotton wool swabs and a suitable antiseptic lotion—e.g. Hibitane aqueous solution 1 in 5000—each swab being used once and then discarded; the labia are separated, the nurse using the fingers of her left hand, to reveal the urethral opening, which is also cleaned. The catheter is held 5–7·5 cms. from the "eye", using either a gauze swab or a pair of forceps, and gently inserted, up to 5 cms., into the urethra. The other end of the catheter is allowed to rest in the receiver. Once urine begins to flow, a specimen may be obtained in a sterile container. If a self-retaining catheter is

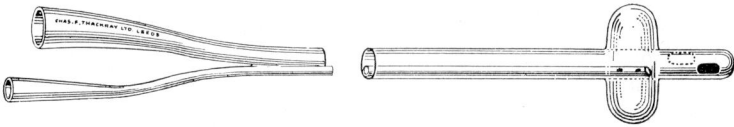

FIG. 35—Foley's catheter. (Approx. $\frac{3}{8}$ sc.).

being used, the appropriate amount (marked on the catheter) of sterile water is injected into the side arm; it may be necessary to tie this with thread. If the catheter is to be removed after obtaining a specimen, it is gently withdrawn and the patient left dry, warm and comfortable. Following catheterisation, many patients feel the need to pass urine even when the bladder has been emptied, and this should be explained to them. If the catheter is to be left in, it is either closed with a sterile spigot or connected by sterile tubing to a drainage bottle. In either case the patient will be more comfortable if the catheter is lightly strapped to the leg so that she is free to move without pulling on the catheter or tubing.

For a male patient, the doctor may require a large-size catheter and a sterile lubricant.

After use, all equipment is cleansed and re-sterilised and disposable equipment is placed in the appropriate bin.

LAVAGE

The word "lavage" is derived from a Latin word "lavo" meaning "to wash", and is used to describe the procedure of washing out a cavity. The equipment needed is basically the same wherever the cavity—i.e. a catheter or special tube, which is connected to a syringe, funnel or special apparatus by means of tubing and

151

connections. The fluid used is often water and is prepared at body temperature; the amount varies according to the size of the cavity and the amount necessary to clean it; it is important that all the fluid used is returned and for this reason known quantities should be used and the amount returned estimated. This is only a sterile procedure when the cavity concerned is normally sterile—e.g. the bladder.

Gastric lavage.—This may be used to prepare the patient who is to have gastric surgery, or to empty and irrigate the stomach in cases of suspected poisoning. The best position for the patient is sitting up—but if unconscious, he should be lying on his side; false teeth must be removed, and the bed and patient are protected by waterproof covers; a bucket is placed on the floor nearby.

The tube used is a large-bore stomach tube, which is lubricated and passed through the mouth.

Tubing and funnel are attached and the washout commenced by filling the funnel with water and allowing it to run into the stomach. Before the funnel is completely empty it is inverted over the bucket, so syphoning back the water and the stomach contents. The lavage is continued in this way until clear fluid is returned on 2 to 3 consecutive occasions. Several litres may have to be used.

In cases of suspected poisoning, all fluid returned is sent to the laboratory for analysis and it is sometimes necessary to save the first specimen separately. The containers are labelled with the patient's name, the date, time and the ward or department. On completing the procedure the nurse withdraws the empty tube and offers a mouthwash to the patient (if conscious). The apparatus is cleared away and the tube sterilised.

Rectal lavage.—This is not so common today, as many physicians and surgeons consider that the use of suppositories is an adequate method of clearing the lower bowel prior to examination or operation. However, if necessary, an enema is given and the rectum is then washed out with water, using similar equipment and employing syphonage to facilitate the return of the fluid. The position of the patient is as for an enema and it is important that he is comfortable since this can be a lengthy procedure.

The term "colonic lavage" is used to indicate cleaning of the colon rather than the rectum and it is rarely carried out except in special hospitals and clinics. The principles are exactly the same as for a rectal washout, but larger quantities of fluid are used and special equipment may be available.

GASTRIC ANALYSIS

One of the functions of the stomach is to secrete hydrochloric acid, which assists in digestion. In certain disorders, the amount may be increased, diminished or there may be an achlorhydria (absence of acid). To assess the amount present, certain tests may be carried out, most of which involve the use of a Ryle's (naso-gastric) tube.

Fractional test meal.—Prior to this test, the patient has nothing to eat or drink from midnight; on waking, a naso-gastric tube is passed into the stomach, and the contents aspirated by attaching a syringe to the free end of the tube. This specimen is put into a labelled container and is usually described as the "fasting" or "resting juice". Some form of meal is then given, to stimulate the cells of the stomach to secrete hydrochloric acid; this may be 50 mls. of 7% alcohol, 300 mls of thin gruel or as ordered. Serial specimens of approximately 5 mls. of gastric contents are then withdrawn and placed in numbered containers at either 15- or 30- minute intervals, for a set period of time, e.g. 2 to 3 hours. At the end of this time the stomach is emptied and the final specimen placed in a container marked "residue".

During the test, the nurse may be asked to test one of the early specimens with litmus paper and if the specimen is not acid an injection of 0·25 to 0·5 mgs. of histamine may be ordered and the test continued. When it is completed, the tube is withdrawn, a mouthwash given and the patient offered his breakfast.

Histamine or insulin tests of gastric function.—Variations of the above include those tests involving the injection of either histamine or insulin, in place of the alcohol or gruel given by mouth. The details vary in different hospitals, but in all cases careful observation of the patient is necessary as the drugs may have side-effects. When asked to carry out either of these tests, the nurse must familiarise herself with local practice, and the drugs concerned.

"Tubeless" test meal.—Within recent years it has become possible to determine the presence or absence of hydrochloric acid in the stomach without passing a Ryle's tube. This is a simple test which is much less unpleasant for the patient and which can, if necessary, be performed by him at home. The substances to be taken by mouth by the patient are supplied, together with full instructions, in a pack labelled "Diagnex[1] blue diagnostic test". If hydrochloric acid is present, the substances are changed, absorbed into the blood stream, and finally excreted in the urine. Specimens of urine are therefore collected as per instructions, and sent to the laboratory.

The patient should be warned of the colour change likely in the urine.

RENAL EFFICIENCY TESTS

The functions of the kidneys include the ability to excrete urea and water, and it is therefore possible to test renal efficiency by giving known quantities of these by mouth and examining the urine passed.

Urea concentration test.—The patient is given nothing to eat or drink from midnight. On waking he is asked to pass urine, and the specimen is placed in a container and carefully labelled. Fifteen grammes of urea are mixed with water and the mixture given to the patient to drink.

Three specimens of urine are then collected at hourly intervals and placed in numbered containers; at the end of the test the patient is given his breakfast and the specimens of urine sent to the laboratory. The blood urea must be known before this test and so a specimen of blood will have been taken by the doctor for this purpose. (The normal blood urea is 20 to 40 mgs. %.)

Concentration and dilution test.—The patient is given nothing to drink from midnight. An early morning specimen of urine is obtained and the specific gravity taken and recorded. The patient is given a measured quantity of water (1000 mls.) to drink over a period of 30 minutes. Three urine specimens are then obtained at hourly intervals and the specific gravity noted and recorded. If the kidneys are functioning normally, the early morning specimen will have a high specific gravity (1·020 to 1·030), and at least one of the subsequent specimens will have a low specific gravity (1·000 to 1·010).

[1] Diagnex Blue—E. R. Squibb & Sons Ltd.

24-hour collections of urine.—These may be required to assess the amount of creatinine and electrolytes (sodium, potassium and chloride) in the urine.

Group 2

BLOOD TRANSFUSION

The preparation of the patient and the equipment for this procedure, and the help given to the doctor, are essentially the same as that described for an intravenous infusion (page 136). However, the nurse has additional responsibilities. The reason for these are concerned with the danger to the patient, should incompatible blood be given.

Many blood groups are known, but the main divisions are into groups A, B, AB, and O—the others being subdivisions of these; in this country the majority of people have blood of either groups A or O. In addition, a further factor—the Rhesus factor—must be taken into account: 85% of all people have this factor in their blood, and are therefore described as being Rhesus positive (Rh. +ve); the remaining 15% do not have it, and so are Rhesus negative (Rh. —ve).

The basic principle underlying all transfusions is that a patient must be given blood of his own group and Rhesus compatibility. Because of this, prior to any transfusion, the doctor takes a sample of the patient's blood, to discover his group; the serum is then re-checked against every bottle of blood to be given—this process being called cross-matching.

The following practical points must be borne in mind: the bottles of blood are stored in refrigerators, which are controlled at a set temperature (ward refrigerators are not suitable); they are removed about $\frac{1}{2}$ hour before being used, and should then remain at room temperature until the blood is given and should not be warmed in any way. It is important that both nurse and doctor check that the blood bottle bears the patient's name, number, ward and date, and that the group corresponds with that recorded in the patient's notes.

While the transfusion is in progress, the patient's condition must be observed closely, and any signs of suspected incompatibility reported at once to the ward sister. These include headache, backache and shivering or rigor; late signs include haematuria and jaundice. Occasionally the reaction is simply due to the introduction of a foreign protein—particularly in patients receiving several transfusions; if this is the case, the doctor may order an antihistamine drug to be given. It is usual to give 600 mls. of blood over a period of 4 to 6 hours unless a quicker transfusion is required.

Most hospitals have their own rules as to the procedure to be adopted when a second or subsequent bottle of blood is put up; in any case, two nurses should be present when the bottles are changed, and should check the label.

When the transfusion is complete, the bottles are returned, unwashed, to the laboratory.

LUMBAR PUNCTURE

Cerebro-spinal fluid is a watery fluid which surrounds the brain and spinal cord in the sub-arachnoid space, and is also found in the ventricles of the brain. It is continually being formed from blood and re-absorbed back into the circulation. Its composition and pressure may be altered in disorders affecting the brain, the spinal cord or their coverings—the meninges. Because of this, specimens are often obtained for diagnostic purposes, and to do this a lumbar puncture is performed. This procedure is also carried out to introduce:

(*a*) Contrast media prior to X-rays (page 100).

(*b*) Anaesthetic substances.

(*c*) Antibiotics.

This is a sterile procedure and a trolley is prepared containing the necessary equipment, which includes swabs and lotions for cleaning the skin, syringes, a local anaesthetic and the lumbar puncture "set"—needles and a manometer. Specimen bottles and laboratory forms should also be available.

The most common position for the patient is the left lateral, and he is asked to bend his head forward and to bring his knees up to his chest. This has the effect of separating the spines of the vertebrae, which makes the introduction of the needle easier. The patient's back should be level with the edge of the bed, and his night wear and bedclothes arranged so that his lumbar region is exposed. An alternative position is to have the patient sitting up, with his head bent forward towards his knees.

The doctor gives a local anaesthetic, and inserts the needle between the 3rd and 4th lumbar vertebrae, as it is here that a specimen of cerebro-spinal fluid may be obtained without risk of damage to the spinal cord, which ends at the level of the

FIG. 36.—Lumbar Puncture Set.

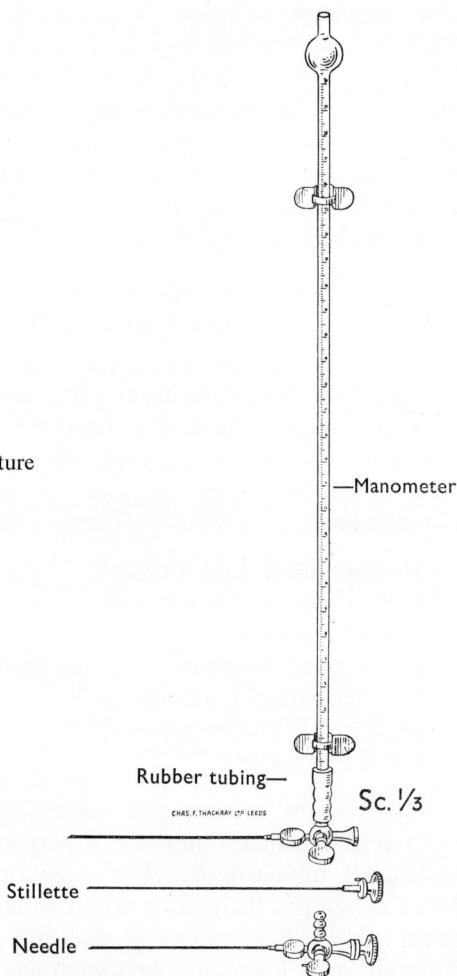

—Manometer

Rubber tubing—

CHAS. F. THACKRAY LTD LEEDS

Sc. ⅓

Stillette

Needle

1st–2nd lumbar vertebrae. During the procedure the nurse supports the patient and assists the doctor if necessary: she may be asked to hold the specimen bottles while fluid is being collected, or to compress the patient's jugular vein while the doctor is checking the pressure of the fluid in the manometer.

After the procedure the patient is made comfortable, and

asked to lie quietly with only one pillow for a period of time—this is to prevent headache, which sometimes follows a lumbar puncture.

The equipment is cleared away, returned to the C.S.S.D., or cleaned and re-sterilised.

A variation of this is the cisternal puncture, when a similar needle (marked in centimetres) is introduced into the cisterna magna at the base of the brain, through the space between the occiput and the atlas vertebra. The preparation of the patient may include shaving the back of his neck, and he is asked to flex his head so that his chin is on his chest. Other details are as before.

REMOVAL OF FLUID

As a result of infection, or disturbance of the circulation of blood and tissue fluid, collections of pus or excess fluid may form in the tissue spaces or in cavities lined by serous membranes.

In the case of oedema (excess fluid in the tissue spaces), various measures can be employed to relieve the condition. These include:

(1) Restriction of fluid intake.
(2) Restriction of salt in the diet.
(3) Use of diuretics.
(4) Mechanical means of removing fluid:
    (*a*) Abdominal paracentesis.
    (*b*) Use of Southey's tubes.
    (*c*) Acu puncture.

If fluid collects between the layers of the pleura, a chest aspiration (paracentesis thoracis) is performed.

Abdominal paracentesis.—The preparation of the patient includes offering a bedpan or urinal to insure that the bladder is empty; this is most important, as a full bladder rises into the abdominal cavity and could be punctured during the procedure. The patient is made comfortable in the sitting position, and a many-tailed bandage may be placed behind him so that the strips can be brought round the abdomen when necessary.

The equipment must be sterile, and includes swabs and lotions for cleaning the skin, syringes and a local anaesthetic, a trocar and cannula, fine tubing which fits the cannula and a

158

Winchester-type bottle into which the fluid will drain. A gate clip is also necessary to control the rate of flow.

The doctor cleans the skin, gives a local anaesthetic and inserts the trocar and cannula; some doctors make a small incision with a scalpel before inserting the trocar. The site of the puncture is commonly mid-way between the umbilicus and the iliac crest. The trocar is removed and the fluid drains down the tubing into the bottle at a steady rate. The cannula is held in position by strapping and the many-tailed bandage fastened firmly across the abdomen; the equipment is cleared away as before. While the fluid is draining, the nurse must observe the patient carefully, as too rapid a withdrawal of fluid may result in collapse; the bandage is gradually adjusted as the girth of the abdomen becomes less, to help support the abdominal contents as the intra-abdominal pressure drops.

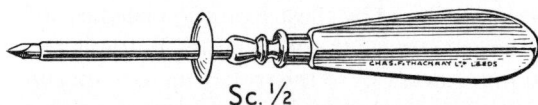

Sc. ½

FIG. 37.—Trocar and Cannula.

The basic care of the patient must be continued as the fluid may drain for several hours. On completion, the cannula is withdrawn, a sterile dressing applied, the bandage removed and the fluid measured and recorded. The dressing is renewed when necessary as further slight leakage may continue for some time.

Insertion of Southey's tubes.—These are fine, perforated silver tubes which may be used to drain excess fluid from the legs. The procedure is similar to that described above, except that no bandage is required. Several pieces of capillary tubing will be needed, and local anaesthetic may take the form of a surface spray, or not be used at all. Several tubes are inserted into each leg by means of an introducer: the patient is nursed in the sitting position, and if possible the bottom part of the bed is lowered.

Acu-puncture.—Occasionally, fluid from the legs is removed through incisions or punctures in the lower part of the legs, or the dorsum of the feet. Once the incisions have been made, the legs are wrapped in sterile towels which need changing frequently. For the patient, this is often a cold, wet and uncomfortable procedure; he can be helped by constant changing of linen and by support and encouragement from the staff. This treatment should not be confused with a long-established Chinese treatment of the same name.

Chest aspiration.—The patient usually sits up, and leans forward with his arms and head resting on a pillow placed on a bed table in front of him: this position has the effect of widening the intercostal spaces. Although one side of the chest must be exposed, the patient should be kept warm. If he has a troublesome cough, a linctus may be given prior to the procedure, as he will be asked to co-operate by not coughing while the needle is in position. It can be explained to him that his breathing will be easier once the fluid is removed.

The equipment needed is sterile and is similar to that required for an abdominal paracentesis, except that the trocar, cannula and tubing are replaced by chest aspiration needles, a 2- or 3-way tap and a large syringe: the Winchester bottle is replaced by a graduated jug. Additions to the trolley include specimen bottles, a laboratory form and sometimes antibiotic substances which are introduced after the fluid has been withdrawn.

During the procedure the nurse supports the patient. The doctor, after cleaning the skin, gives a local anaesthetic and inserts the needle between the layers of the pleura. Care is taken not to introduce air, and for this reason a 2-way tap is used while the fluid is being withdrawn. The nurse may be asked to hold the specimen bottles or jug. When the needle is withdrawn, the puncture is sealed with collodion or a sterile dressing applied. The patient is made comfortable, and the equipment cleared away. The procedure is basically the same if air is to be removed—i.e. following a pneumothorax.

BONE MARROW PUNCTURE

In certain suspected blood disorders, it is necessary to obtain a specimen of red bone marrow as this will give more detailed information as to the development and formation of new blood cells than can be obtained from a blood sample. The bone used is usually the sternum, except in the case of small children when the crest of the tibia may be used.

As has already been mentioned, it is necessary to give a careful explanation before all procedures: in this instance it is especially important since during the procedure the patient may experience an unpleasant feeling of pressure; true pain, however, is not usually felt.

The patient lies on his back, with one pillow, and with the front of the chest exposed.

The equipment is sterile, and includes swabs and lotions for cleaning the skin, local anaesthetic, a syringe, a marrow puncture needle with a guard attached, and glass slides.

The laboratory will provide special containers for the specimens. The doctor cleans the skin, gives the local anaesthetic, sets the guard at the correct place and inserts the needle; a specimen is then obtained, the needle withdrawn and a sterile dressing applied. The nurse supports the patient during the procedure and makes him comfortable afterwards.

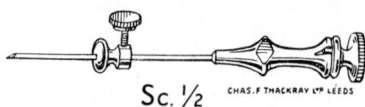

Fig. 38.—Marrow Puncture Needle.

The equipment is cleared away.

Group 3

ESTIMATION OF THE BASAL METABOLIC RATE (B.M.R.)

The Basal Metabolic Rate (page 60) is altered in certain disorders of the thyroid gland: it can be estimated by measuring a patient's oxygen consumption and carbon dioxide output, and correlating these in relation to his height, weight and skin surface area.

This test must be performed when the patient is at rest, and is therefore best done first thing in the morning. A careful explanation is given the night before, and after a good night's sleep the patient is left undisturbed until the technician arrives to carry out the test. If desired, a bedpan or urinal is given, but the patient should not be allowed out of bed and is not given any medicines unless ordered. When the test is finished, he is able to wash, have his breakfast and carry on with normal routine. Because of the preparation necessary it is advisable to have the patient in a side room. Many physicians now think that this test is only of value if 2 to 3 estimations are made.

ENDOSCOPY

Direct examination of a body cavity is called endoscopy, and the instruments used are endoscopes. These are rigid or semi-rigid hollow tubes containing a lens system; as the cavities to be examined are inside the body, a lighting system is provided in the form of a bulb, flex and battery. It is usual to refer to a specific examination by using as prefix a name referring to the cavity to be examined, e.g.:

bronchoscopy (bronchoscope)—examination of the bronchi;
gastroscopy (gastroscope)—examination of the stomach;
sigmoidoscopy (sigmoidoscope)—examination of the sigmoid colon;
proctoscopy (proctoscope)—examination of the rectum;
cystoscopy (cystoscope)—examination of the bladder.

The preparation for most of these may include the preparation and after-care of a patient who is having a general anaesthetic (see Chapter XII); however, it is usual for adult patients to have a local anaesthetic or, in the case of examination of the lower bowel—no anaesthetic at all.

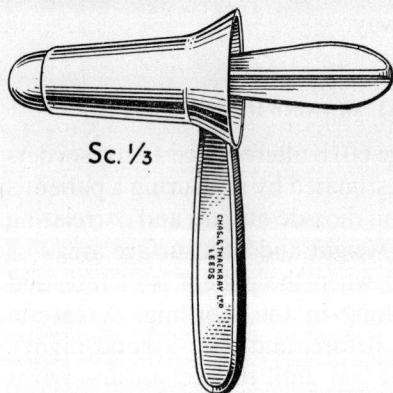

Sc. ⅓

FIG. 39.—Proctoscope.

Bronchoscopy and gastroscopy.—The preparation of the patient, and his after-care, is similar for both these: 1 to 1½ hours prior to the examination he is dressed in a theatre gown, his dentures are removed and a pre-medication is given. This usually consists of a sedative and an anti-secretory drug: if a local anaesthetic is to be used, anaesthetic lozenges are given to the patient to suck. These examinations are usually carried out in the theatre.

On his return to the ward it is important that he is given nothing to eat or drink for several hours, as his cough and

162

swallowing reflexes will be absent until the effect of the local anaesthetic wears off.

Sigmoidoscopy and proctoscopy.—As these are examinations of the lower bowel, some preparation to clear the area of faeces may be ordered.

Both may be performed in the ward, and they are not sterile procedures. Although they are not painful examinations, the patient may feel some discomfort. The proctoscope is a small instrument which is normally part of ward equipment and may or may not have a battery and light attached; a lubricant and swabs should be provided.

If the examinations are performed in theatre, the normal preparation is carried out.

Cystoscopy.—This is performed in theatre and a light anaesthetic is usually given, and the preparation for this and the after-care of the patient is as described in Chapter XII. This examination is necessary if a retrograde pyelogram is to be carried out (page 99).

Chapter XI

FURTHER NURSING CARE AND WARD EMERGENCIES

On admission to hospital, the patient is usually taken to the ward specialising in the treatment that he will need. It follows that both wards and patients tend to be classified as "medical", "surgical", "gynaecological", etc. In the newer hospitals patients may be grouped according to the intensity of treatment and nursing care required, i.e. in intensive, intermediate and minimal care units. However, all patients need the same basic nursing care, understanding and support outlined in the early chapters of this book, plus any particular treatment required for the specific condition.

The "medical" patient is often in hospital for a longer period than his "surgical" counterpart, and the results of his treatment are not always so obvious; many medical conditions become chronic over a period of years and the patient may visit the same hospital and ward on several different occasions.

There is a pattern of care for all patients, which involves rest, modification of diet where necessary, the use of various drugs, sometimes surgery and often advice to the patient to adopt certain modifications to his way of life.

REST

To ensure adequate rest it is necessary not only to attend to the patient's general needs but to see that the affected part is also rested. The way in which this is achieved depends on the system in question; for example, a patient with a peptic ulcer has small, frequent, regular meals to rest his stomach, whereas a patient with a fracture may have a plaster-of-paris splint applied in order to rest the limb. In some cases the patient must be nursed at "complete rest". This means that he is not allowed to do anything for himself; he is washed and fed by the nursing staff, lifted on and off bedpans and all his needs attended to. For a normally active person this can be extremely trying, especially when he is not feeling particularly ill. Great encouragement is necessary and some form of mental stimulus should be

164

provided whenever possible; this may be in the form of radio, television or frequent visitors. The nurse can also help the patient to keep up to date by reading newspapers to him. As his condition improves, he is gradually allowed to do more for himself, over a period of time. This regimen is usually ordered for patients with severe heart disease—e.g. coronary thrombosis, or in those conditions which may lead to heart damage if untreated—e.g. rheumatic fever.

Modification of diet.—See page 68.

Uses of drugs.—See page 113.

Surgery.—The preparation of a patient for theatre and his care afterwards are discussed in the next chapter.

REHABILITATION

The rehabilitation of the patient must start as soon as the acute phase of his illness is over—which may be a day or two after admission—and may continue for many months after his discharge. Several members of the hospital team will help, including the medical social worker, occupational therapist and physiotherapist, and if necessary their work will be continued by their colleagues in the local authority services. For those left with any disability it is often possible to obtain help through various agencies, including the Disablement Resettlement Officer. This part of the patient's treatment is as important as his basic nursing care, and in fact may form part of it; for example, the nursing care of a patient suffering from diabetes mellitus includes teaching him to check and administer his own insulin, to test his own urine and to understand the modifications necessary in his diet.

CARE OF THE UNCONSCIOUS PATIENT

The care of the unconscious patient demands the highest standards of basic nursing and observation, since the patient is not in a position to communicate his needs to the nurse.

The airway.—The patient is usually nursed in the semi-prone position to ensure a clear airway. If excessive secretions collect in his mouth, these should be removed by suction; a small tray should be prepared and placed on the locker, containing a mouth gag and tongue forceps. These may be necessary should the patient's airway become obstructed due to the tongue slipping back.

In some cases an artificial airway is made into the trachea—that is, a tracheostomy is performed; this must also be kept clear.

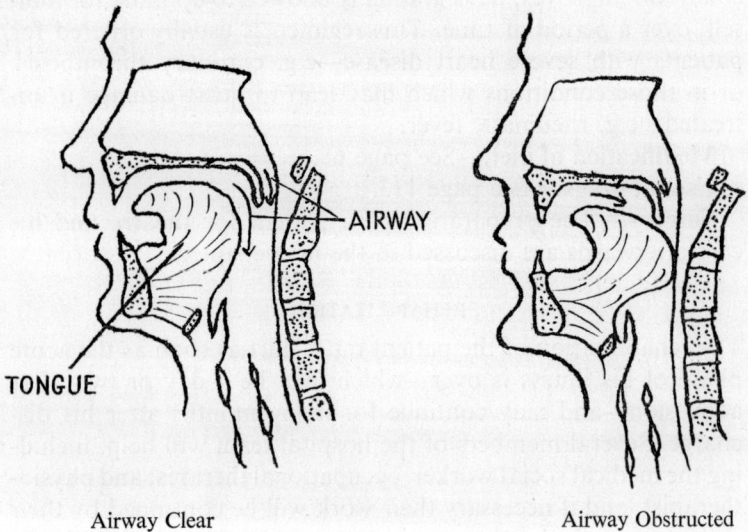

Airway Clear   Airway Obstructed

FIG. 40.

General nursing care.—The patient should be given a daily blanket bath and his face and hands sponged at intervals throughout the day: special attention must be paid to those areas of the body where 2 skin surfaces are in apposition. When the patient has been washed, his hair should be brushed and combed; in the case of a woman with long hair, it must be kept free of tangles and may be easier to control if tied back with a ribbon.

The patient must be turned at least 2-hourly, partly to prevent the occurrence of pressure sores and partly to facilitate full expansion of both lungs. Since he is not eating or drinking, his mouth must be cleaned 4-hourly or when necessary, to prevent dryness and cracking of the mucous membranes. In many cases it is necessary to clean his eyes regularly, using cotton wool swabs and water, or normal saline, and to instil a drop of oil—e.g. parolein—into each, to keep the surface of the eye moist; the unconscious patient tends to lie with his eyes partly open, and as the blink reflex is absent, the surface becomes unduly dry.

Feeding and fluid balance.—If the patient is unconscious for a prolonged period, a naso-gastric tube is passed and intra-gastric feeding started (page 134). The patient's needs are less than normal, as his activity is minimal, and a special fluid diet will be worked out by the dietitian or ward sister to provide approximately 2000 calories a day, an adequate fluid intake and the necessary food factors. A fluid-balance chart must be kept to ensure an accurate record.

Bladder and bowels.—A self-retaining catheter is usually passed into the bladder, which is kept empty, either by removing the spigot at 4-hourly intervals, or by continuous drainage. The output is recorded and the urine tested daily.

To prevent constipation and/or faecal incontinence, an enema or suppository may be given every 2 to 3 days.

Exercises.—The patient's limbs must be exercised each time the bed is made or nursing care given; as well as this, the physiotherapist will carry out the full range of passive movements of each limb daily.

Hazards.—The unconscious patient is prone to all the complications which can occur in those confined to bed, and in addition he cannot complain if he is too hot, too cold or if he is placed in an unnatural or an uncomfortable position.

Observations.—The observations to be made include many already mentioned—e.g. state of the skin, eyes and mouth, plus his colour, temperature, pulse and respiration rates and his level of consciousness. This last can be assessed by noting his reaction to stimuli—i.e. his response when spoken to, or when being moved, and by testing his eyes for pupil reaction and size. Normally the pupils are equal and react to strong light by contracting. The blood pressure is taken and recorded at intervals as ordered by the doctor—this may range from $\frac{1}{4}$-hourly to once daily. It is important that any change in the patient's condition is reported immediately.

CARE OF THE PARALYSED PATIENT

The total care of the paralysed patient depends on the extent of his disability and the part affected. The term hemiplegia (hemiparesis) means paralysis of one side of the body, as seen follow-

167

ing a cerebral vascular accident (stroke), and paraplegia—paralysis below the waist. An important part of the patient's care is his rehabilitation—that is, helping him to regain independence. An added complication in some cases of hemiplegia is dysphasia—that is, the speech centre is affected and the patient is unable to communicate; this is extremely distressing to both the patient and his relatives, and the nurse must remember that in most cases his intelligence is unimpaired, and his hearing normal. The feelings of one such patient are admirably described in *Stroke*, by Douglas Ritchie, which the nurse is advised to read.

General care.—The general nursing care is much the same as that provided for the unconscious patient, except that many

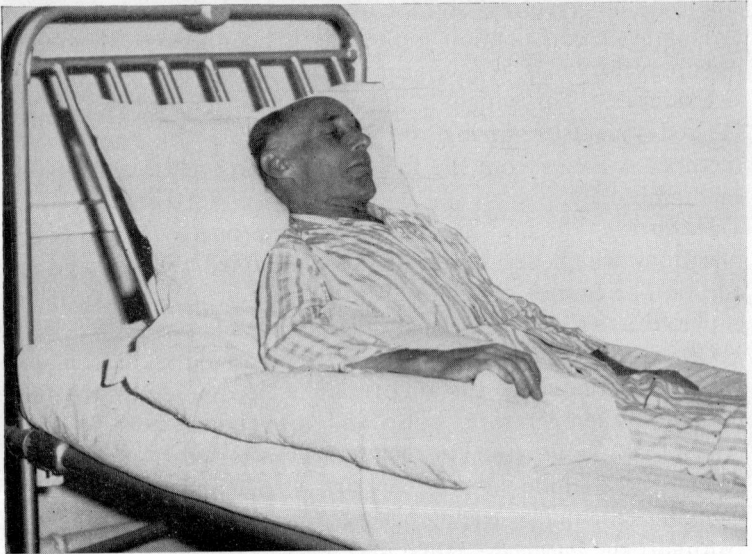

FIG. 41.—Position of Paralysed Hand and Arm.

paralysed patients can eat and drink normally—sometimes with help—and most are able to maintain their own airway.

Position.—The position of the paralysed limbs is extremely important to minimise the risk of deformities. The position of the leg(s) is maintained by the careful placing of pillows and foot-boards, with the knee in slight flexion. A cradle should be used to prevent pressure from the bedclothes. The arm is supported, and a sponge or cotton wool roll place in the hand with the thumb and fingers in apposition.

Movements.—The paralysed limbs are put through the full range of passive movement 3 to 4 times a day, and as soon as possible active movements are encouraged.

Care of the bladder and bowels.—For those patients with paraplegia, a further problem is re-education of the bladder. Tone is maintained by emptying the bladder at regular intervals, either by releasing the spigot in a catheter every 4 hours, or by offering bedpans or urinals at regular intervals and encouraging the patient to use them. It may take months before control is achieved. The bowels may be controlled by the use of suppositories.

Observations.—These include the state of the skin and paralysed limbs, including the warmth of the extremities, the state of the bladder and bowels and any improvement in movement or sensation of the affected part.

Since the patient is often left with a permanent disability he must be encouraged to do things for himself, and made aware of the facilities and help available to him when he leaves hospital.

CARE OF THE INFECTIOUS PATIENT

Even in general hospitals it is sometimes necessary to isolate a patient so that he is not a danger to other patients in the ward. The infectious diseases such as measles are not often seen, except in a children's ward, but patients may be isolated for such conditions as dysentery, tuberculosis or wound infection. This method of nursing is called barrier nursing or isolation nursing, and the details of the way in which it is carried out vary considerably from one hospital to another, but the principles on which they are based are the same. If the routes by which infection is spread are understood, a technique can easily be worked out (page 110).

Ideally, the patient should be nursed in a side room or cubicle with a washbasin, near to the sanitary annexes. If this is not possible, a corner bed should be used. Sometimes screens are placed round the bed, but if this is done it must be realised that the screens in no way form a barrier but are merely a reminder to the nurse.

Crockery and cutlery.—Nowadays, the introduction of disposable crockery and cutlery has simplified this aspect of barrier nursing. The articles are used once, and then disposed of, by burning: this greatly lessens the risk of cross-infection.

An older method is to boil all utensils for 5 minutes after a meal, before placing them with the rest of the crockery. Waste food should be placed in a suitable container—e.g. a paper bag —and burnt.

Linen.—All personal and bed linen should be placed in a special marked bag, or bin and sent separately to the hospital laundry.

Bedpans, urinals and excreta.—It is not always necessary to take special measures when dealing with excreta; however, in some cases where infection is carried in the urine and faeces, e.g. typhoid fever, disinfection must be carried out. The contents of the bedpan or urinal are covered with a suitable disinfectant, and left for 2 hours before being emptied in the usual way.

Clinical thermometers.—No added precautions are necessary, since each patient has his own thermometer, which is normally kept in an antiseptic solution.

Uses of gowns and masks.—It is customary for medical and nursing staff to wear a gown when attending to the patient; a mask is worn if necessary—i.e. in airborne infections such as pulmonary tuberculosis. The use of overshoes is becoming more common. Gowns and masks should be available near the patient's bed and the gowns should be changed every 24 hours or when soiled. Care should be taken when putting on a gown —the outside must be regarded as contaminated.

Before and after attending to a patient and before finally leaving the area, all staff must wash and dry their hands; a plentiful supply of hand towels—preferably paper—and hand cream must be available. The use of disposable equipment has made barrier nursing technique much easier and lessened the risk of cross-infection.

General care.—The care given will vary with the condition of the patient, and will depend on his symptoms: basically, it will be the same as for any patient confined to bed. The reasons for the precautions being taken should be explained.

Some patients will not enjoy being isolated, and a radio or some other interest should be provided; as a rule, visitors are allowed.

Terminal disinfection.—When precautions are no longer necessary, or the patient goes home, all equipment must be disinfected in the way described, before being returned to general use. The room is aired, and the furniture, walls and floors washed and/or polished.

Minor accidents happen within the hospital to both patients and staff. The "first aid" is not quite the same as in the home, since full hospital facilities are immediately available. It is also helpful for the nurse to know what to do in certain emergencies since there will be occasions when she is the only person at hand.

Fainting.—A faint is due to a sudden fall in blood pressure, causing a decrease in the amount of blood circulating in the cerebral vessels. The cause of this may be shock due to injury or emotion, immobility in an upright position and such simple things as a hot stuffy atmosphere and sudden exertion on an empty stomach. In the ward, patients who have been confined to bed for long periods may feel faint when getting up for the first time and some may complain of faintness in the bath, especially if the water is too hot. The person who faints, falls to the floor, is pale, the skin feels cold and the pulse is slow. Until he regains consciousness he should be left lying flat, since this is the best position for maintaining the blood supply to the vital centres, especially the brain. In most cases the period of unconsciousness is very short.

Treatment consists of loosening tight clothing, ensuring a plentiful supply of fresh air and, in the case of a patient, getting him back to bed as soon as possible, i.e. when he is conscious and help is available. Should a patient faint when in the sitting position and be unable to fall, he should be laid flat either on the floor or in bed. If this is impossible, for example if it occurs in a confined space, his head should be lowered to between his knees. The faint should be reported to the nurse in charge together with any observations made at the time. Unless contra-indicated, a hot drink is given to the patient, and he is kept under careful observation.

Cuts.—Nurses occasionally cut themselves when handling broken glass equipment, e.g. glass connections or ampoules. The cut should be rinsed under cold running water, a dry dress-

171

ing applied and the incident reported. All accidents to staff or patients must be recorded on the appropriate form or in the accident book. It is important that this is done as soon as possible after the incident.

Burns and scalds.—The only difference between a burn and a scald is the causative agent; a burn is caused by dry heat and a scald by moist heat. The injury produced may be simple reddening of the skin, blistering or destruction of skin and underlying tissues. The emergency care is to cover the area with a dry dressing and if necessary to treat for shock. If the burn is due to chemicals—e.g. lysol—the area should be irrigated, using running water, and covered with a dressing. The incident must be reported.

Epistaxis, or bleeding from the nose.—This is a fairly common event and in many cases is of short duration and produces few ill-effects. The victim should sit down, preferably near an open window, and pressure should be applied just below the bridge of the nose. In the majority of cases this treatment is effective and the bleeding stops. If necessary a cold compress can be applied to the area, and it is advisable to warn the patient not to blow his nose until bleeding has ceased for several minutes. Rarely, the bleeding continues and medical aid must then be sought.

Haematemesis (Haem—blood, emesis—vomiting).—This may be due to peptic ulcer, oesophageal varices or a patient may vomit blood which he has previously swallowed. The emergency treatment is to lie the patient down, reassure him and send for a doctor. A mouthwash is refreshing, but nothing should be given to drink. The vomit should be saved, if possible, for inspection by the sister and doctor, the nurse should stay with the patient until relieved and should note his colour, pulse rate and any restlessness or complaints of pain or discomfort.

Haemoptysis.—This is the term used to describe coughing up blood from the lungs. The amounts are usually much smaller than in haematemesis and the blood looks frothy since it is mixed with air. The patient is placed in a comfortable position in which he can breathe easily and is reassured. The doctor is informed and the observations made by the nurse are as those described in haematemesis. The patient is advised to cough as little as possible.

Ruptured varicose vein of leg.—An injury to a superficial varicose vein may produce sudden profuse bleeding; with prompt treatment the patient will suffer few ill-effects, but if treatment is delayed for any reason, a large quantity of blood may be lost and the patient become shocked. The immediate treatment is to sit or lie the patient down, support and elevate the affected limb and apply direct pressure to the bleeding point. This is best achieved by bandaging a clean pad firmly in position. The doctor is informed.

Fits.—When someone has a fit he becomes unconscious, falls to the ground and convulsive movements occur in various parts of the body. The patient may become cyanosed and be incontinent. The dangers are that he may injure himself in falling or that the airway may become obstructed. The emergency treatment is to remove any obvious hazard and to try to maintain an efficient airway by keeping the patient's head turned to one side, but his movements should not be restricted in any other way. Observations should be made as to the duration of the fit and the parts of the body affected. When he recovers consciousness, he may be rather dazed and should be assisted to his bed, where he will probably fall into a deep sleep.

Falls.—If a patient falls out of bed, or slips while he is up in the ward, the incident must be reported immediately. If necessary the nurse should get help and assist, or lift, the patient back to bed. Any obvious injury or complaint of pain or discomfort should be noted and reported to the doctor, when he arrives to examine him. As mentioned before, all accidents are entered in a book kept for this purpose.

Chapter XII

PRE- AND POST-OPERATIVE CARE

Routine work and nursing care in a surgical ward are rather more dramatic than in a medical ward. The average length of stay for each patient is short and most patients get up within a day or two of their operation and need little detailed nursing care after the first few days. Surgeons nowadays tend to concentrate on surgery of one region of the body, with the result that surgical nursing has now become subdivided into many specialities. However, the preparation of the patient for theatre, his care afterwards and many of the complications which may arise, are basically the same wherever the site of operation; once the principles of care have been learned, they can be applied in any surgical ward.

PRE-OPERATIVE CARE

This can be divided into the psychological and physical preparation of the patient.

Psychological preparation.—Whether it is apparent or not, the majority of patients worry about their forthcoming operation, especially if it is a mutilating one, e.g. removal of a limb (amputation) or of a breast (mastectomy). To overcome this, explanations, varying with the intelligence and emotional state of the patient, must be given, preferably by the surgeon in charge. Even when this has been done, many patients need constant reassurance and support from the nursing staff, who must never forget that what to them is a routine daily occurrence is a major event in the patient's life.

Apart from the patient's own worries, the relatives must be considered, and they should be interviewed by a senior member of the nursing staff; in the course of conversation it may be obvious that there are financial or social difficulties—these should be referred to the ward sister, and through her to the medical social worker.

Other major fears, for many, are concerned with the anaesthetic, but these can be overcome, or even avoided, by simple explanations regarding the premedication and what will happen in the anaesthetic room; it is often reassuring for the patient to realise that one of the ward staff will stay with him until he is asleep—and will be there when he regains consciousness. If the patient wishes to see his priest or minister, arrangements should be made.

Physical preparation.—Before operation, all patients are examined by the house surgeon, and any routine tests, such as X-rays or blood tests, are carried out. It is also usual for the anaesthetist to visit the patient the day before, to assess his fitness for the anaesthetic and to explain it to him. The patient's written consent is necessary in all cases, for both the operation and the anaesthetic, and the nurse must see that the appropriate form is signed. If the patient is under 18, it must be signed by the parent or guardian or the next of kin.

Preparations for surgery may extend over several days beforehand in certain cases. Following admission, the patient's urine is tested in the ward, and the result recorded: any abnormalities must be reported to the house surgeon.

Any exercises which are to be carried out post-operatively, e.g. breathing exercises or leg movements, should be explained, taught and practised. It is advisable for heavy smokers to cut down, or even stop smoking for 2 to 3 days before the anaesthetic; when chest surgery is to be carried out, this may be for a longer period.

It is not customary for suppositories or an enema to be given before every operation, but this is often a routine preparation for surgery of the alimentary tract or pelvic organs; the surgeon's wishes should be ascertained. If some such procedure is ordered, it is usually carried out the day before.

Most patients are given a normal diet to within a few hours of surgery. It is, however, most important that nothing is given to eat or drink within 6 hours of the anaesthetic. It is often a routine to fast patients from midnight the night before, but this is only satisfactory for those patients going to theatre in the early part of the morning. If the theatre list is a long one, those patients at the end should be given a light early breakfast. Before operations on the alimentary tract, or on patients with diabetes mellitus, special care is necessary. These dietary alterations or restrictions will be ordered by the doctor and must be carefully carried out.

It is important that the patient has a good night's sleep before the operation, and as he is likely to be apprehensive, a sedative is usually prescribed and given.

The local preparation of the area involved includes shaving the pubic area or axillae, as necessary; cleaning the skin, either by asking the patient to have a bath or, if he is confined to bed, by washing the area with soap and water; or, occasionally, by cleaning the skin with antiseptic solutions as requested by the surgeon. If iodine is to be applied either in the ward or in theatre, a skin test should be carried out to make sure that the patient is not sensitive to this lotion. In a few instances the surgeon may wish the area to be covered with sterile towels following cleansing with an antiseptic.

For patients admitted as surgical emergencies, the local preparation may be carried out in the theatre.

The immediate preparation includes the removal of all jewellery, hair clips, make up and dentures, and dressing the patient in a suitable open-backed gown, and perhaps a theatre cap and socks. If the site of operation is above the waist, pyjama trousers or briefs may be left on.

Just before giving the pre-medication, the patient is offered a bedpan or urinal, to make sure that the bladder is empty. For certain low abdominal or pelvic operations a catheter may be inserted and left in position. Prior to operations on the gastro-intestinal tract, a naso-gastric tube may be passed into the stomach and left in position.

The pre-medication is given $\frac{1}{2}$ to $1\frac{1}{2}$ hours before the scheduled time of operation. This consists of 2 or more drugs, usually given by injection (hypodermic or intramuscular), which sedate the patient, and prevent formation of secretions. The effects of these drugs should be explained to the patient, as it will not be possible for him to have a drink when his mouth becomes dry. The patient is left to rest quietly until it is time for him to go to theatre. He is then lifted gently on to the trolley and accompanied to theatre by a nurse who carries his notes, X-rays and anything else required.

It sometimes happens that the theatre list is changed at the last minute, and it is therefore important for the nurse to tell the anaesthetist if, when and how the pre-medication was given.

176

POST-OPERATIVE CARE

While the patient is in theatre, his bed is re-made, using clean linen, the top bedclothes being arranged as a pack and the head of the bed being protected by a dressing mackintosh and towel. If waterproof sheeting is not placed under the bottom sheet as routine, the nurse should check this point, as the patient may be confined to bed for 2 or 3 days. Pillows and any other accessories likely to be needed are placed on a nearby chair. Special apparatus, such as oxygen and suction equipment, is checked, so that it is ready for immediate use if required. A small tray is prepared, containing articles necessary to keep the patient's airway clear. This is commonly called the post-anaesthetic, or recovery tray, and the contents include swabs and swab-holding forceps, tongue forceps, a mouth gag and a vomit bowl. This tray is placed on the patient's locker, or if several patients are to go to theatre, on a table nearby.

On return to the ward, the patient is lifted on to the bed and placed in the semi-prone position, care being taken to ensure that his limbs are not subject to undue pressure; this position helps to maintain a clear airway, as excess secretions will drain out of the mouth instead of trickling back into the air passages and the tongue is kept forward. A metal or rubber airway may be in position in his mouth—this will be ejected as he regains consciousness.

The patient should be under constant observation until he regains consciousness. During the first few hours he is gradually raised to the sitting position, unless this is contraindicated; his hands and face are washed and the operation gown replaced by his own pyjamas or night wear.

Observations to be made during the immediate post-operative period are—the colour, state of the skin, pulse and respiration rates, blood pressure recordings if ordered, state of the dressing, if and when urine is passed, restlessness and any complaints of pain or discomfort. Any unusual observations should be reported. An analgesic is usually given when the patient is restless or in pain—this is prescribed before he leaves the theatre.

If a blood transfusion, or intravenous infusion is in progress, further observations will be made as described for these procedures. If the patient vomits, the amount and type should be

177

recorded, and he should be given a mouthwash. Unless contra-indicated, sips of water may be given when he is conscious, and the amounts gradually increased if no vomiting occurs.

Further care and treatment will depend on the nature of the operation, but for most patients breathing exercises and leg movements should be encouraged, diet is gradually introduced, analgesics are given as required and prescribed, and the patient is sat out of bed as soon as his condition permits.

NOTES ON ANAESTHETICS

Much of the care described above relates to the patient who has had a general anaesthetic, when many reflex centres, e.g. coughing and swallowing, are affected and varying levels of unconsciousness achieved. However, there are occasions when the patient's co-operation is required, or he is unfit for a general anaesthetic, and in these cases it is necessary to use either a local, regional or spinal analgesic.

Local analgesia.—Injections of procaine or one of its derivatives are used to anaesthetise the skin and subcutaneous tissues: a varient of this is surface anaesthesia, commonly used in eye surgery, when cocaine drops are instilled before the patient goes to theatre.

Regional analgesia.—This is a method whereby a region of the body—e.g. the arm—is anaesthetised by injections of procaine or one of its derivatives, into the nerve plexus supplying the region—e.g. the brachial plexus.

Spinal analgesia.—To achieve this a lumbar puncture is performed and a solution of a special procaine derivative is introduced: the type of solution depends on the region of the body to be anaesthetised.

With the above substances the area affected will be insensitive and pain will not be experienced until the effect wears off. The nurse must remember that although the patient is conscious, a type of anaesthetic has been given.

CARE OF THE WOUND

Simple ward dressing.—The intact skin forms a barrier which prevents the entry of micro-organisms. During surgery, an incision is made which breaks this barrier, and techniques must be used to prevent the entry of infection until the wound has healed. This affects the nurse in that whenever she inspects or dresses the wound, aseptic technique must be employed.

A clean stitched wound—that is, a wound with no drainage tubes—is best left covered until the stitches or clips are removed, unless there are indications that the wound is infected. Most wounds are covered with a dry gauze dressing and sealed with Elastoplast. If there is a drainage tube, extra layers of absorbent dressings are applied, and the whole bandaged in position. In recent years, a substance has been produced which can be sprayed on the wound and when dry forms a transparent, waterproof seal: no dressing is then required.

To carry out a simple ward dressing, a trolley is prepared containing the sterile dressings, lotions and forceps required; it is easier and safer if 2 nurses are available for this procedure. The patient is made comfortable in a suitable position, so that the area is exposed. One nurse carries out the dressing, the other acting as her assistant, and both wearing masks.

The assistant's duties are concerned with the preparation of the trolley and handing the sterile equipment to the dresser, using forceps. When the dressing is complete, she clears the trolley, disposes of the soiled dressings and if necessary prepares for the next dressing.

The dresser removes the outer dressing and washes and dries her hands. She returns to the patient and removes the inner dressing with forceps handed to her from the trolley by the assistant—these forceps are then discarded. The assistant hands her fresh forceps and she cleans the wound, using swabs and suitable lotions; the wound is then dried and a fresh dressing applied. The patient is made comfortable and the dresser washes her hands again before proceeding to the next patient. Any discoloration, swelling or discharge noted during the dressing should be reported.

With the introduction of disposable equipment and pre-packed dressings, the above procedure has become much simpler—indeed, the top of the trolley may simply have one pack on it, containing all the necessary sterile equipment. The safest way of disposing of dirty dressings is to place them straight into a paper bag, clipped to the side of the trolley; the bag is removed and placed in the dressing bin to be burned later in the hospital incinerator.

It is impossible to describe a dressing technique that will apply in detail to all hospitals—for example, gowns and paper caps may be worn when doing dressings, and in many hospitals only one nurse may be available.

Care of drainage tubes.—A drainage tube is inserted if a discharge of blood, pus, serum or any other body fluid is expected. The tube is usually made of rubber or plastic and varies in shape, being either corrugated, round or adapted for some special purpose, e.g. a "T" tube. At the end of the operation the tube is often stitched in position through the skin, and instructions will be given as to how long it is to remain in place, or when it is to be shortened.

If round tubing is used, it may be connected to further sterile tubing and allowed to drain into a bottle clipped to, or placed at the side of, the bed; this bottle may contain a measured amount of an antiseptic solution which covers the end of the tube and so prevents ascending infection. Otherwise the tube ends in the dressing, which must be renewed when necessary.

When instructed, the dressing is taken down, the stitch removed, the tubing gently withdrawn and a fresh dressing applied. Alternatively, the stitch is removed, and the drainage tube shortened—that is, it is gently withdrawn for approximately 3 cms, a sterile safety pin is inserted about 1·5 cms from the skin and the tubing beyond this cut off; a piece of gauze is placed around the tube, under the pin, to protect the skin, and a fresh dressing applied.

A "T" tube is one inserted to drain the common bile duct: it is left in for several days and instructions for its management and removal will be given; however, its removal is sometimes uncomfortable for the patient, and an analgesic may be prescribed $\frac{1}{2}$ to 1 hour before.

After removal of any drainage tube, rapid healing occurs unless infection is present.

Special care is necessary when nursing a patient who has an operation involving opening the chest. In this case the drainage tube is connected to further tubing, the end of which is placed in a bottle containing water, which forms an underwater seal. The reason for this is to prevent air being sucked into the chest, so causing collapse of the lung. As the patient breathes, free rise and fall of water may be noted in the last part of the tubing, which is often made of glass. It is important that the bottle is always kept below the level of the patient's chest and in some hospitals the tubing is clamped with forceps whenever nursing care is given to the patient, or the bottle changed.

Packs.—Wounds normally heal by what is called first intention—that is, the edges are stitched together and become joined by fibrous tissue, which is seen as a scar. However, if, as the result of surgery, a cavity is formed, the area may be packed with gauze, so that healing takes place from the bottom outwards over a period of days or sometimes weeks. The pack may be renewed—often in theatre—after the first few days, or gradually removed in much the same way as a drainage tube is shortened.

Removal of stitches and clips.—Suture materials include catgut, silk, linen thread and nylon: catgut is used inside the body and is gradually absorbed—removal being unnecessary; the rest are used mainly for the skin and are removed after several days when healing has taken place. Clips are metal fasteners used on the skin, and on the whole are removed earlier than stitches; sometimes both stitches and clips are used for the same wound.

The time for removal varies with both patient and surgeon, and with the site of the incision, but is commonly 3 to 5 days after operation for clips, and 7 to 10 days for stitches. A trolley is prepared as for a simple ward dressing with the addition of either stitch scissors or clip removers. During the dressing, the stitches to be removed are taken out by holding the cut ends of the stitch with forceps held in the left hand, and cutting the stitch between the knot and the skin with the scissors held in the right hand: it can then be gently removed from the wound. On completion, a fresh dressing is applied. Any abnormality of the wound—redness, discharge or obvious failure of healing—should be reported before removing the stiches, and if after removal the wound gapes a little, a dry dressing is applied and the wound edges pulled together by means of an Elastoplast strip.

The procedure above applies to the commonly used interrupted sutures; the wound may be closed in other ways and if so instructions for removal of the stitches will be given in the ward.

Michel clips are removed with special forceps (see diagram). The clip is steadied with forceps held in the left hand and removed by holding the removers in the right hand, inserting the curved blade under the centre of the clip and pressing the two blades together. This has the effect of straightening the clip

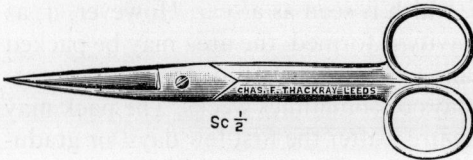

Sc ½

(a) Stitch Scissors.

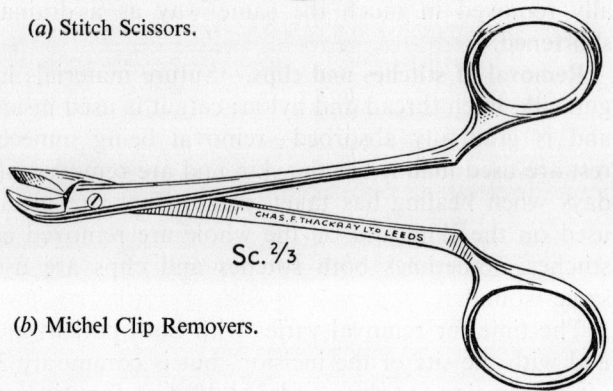

Sc. ²/₃

(b) Michel Clip Removers.

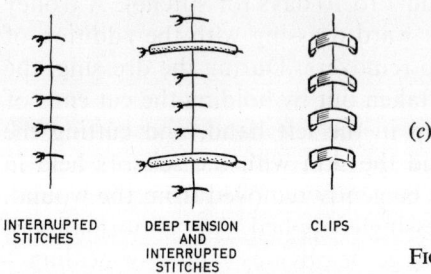

INTERRUPTED STITCHES

DEEP TENSION AND INTERRUPTED STITCHES

CLIPS

(c)

FIG. 42.

and removing the edges from the skin. Care must be taken when lifting it clear as the under-surface of each clip has 2 sharp projections. Observations are made and a clean dressing applied as before.

Kifa clips are removed by pressing the two upper projections together.

Gynaecological procedures.—In a gynaecological ward the

general care of the patient is as described in this chapter. However, since the site of operation may involve the vagina and vulva, special measures are employed to keep these areas clean.

Vulval swabbing.—This is essentially the same procedure as that described prior to catheterisation: a trolley is prepared to contain the necessary sterile swabs, forceps and lotions, and the patient is made comfortable in a suitable position, with a mackintosh and towel under the buttocks. Many different lotions may be used, e.g. Aqueous solution of Hibitane 1 in 5000, and these are prepared at body temperature. The nurse washes her hands, and the area is cleaned, using swabs dipped in the lotion: each swab is used once only and the area cleaned from above downwards. The vulva is then dried carefully and any perineal stitches may be dabbed with spirit; a sterile pad is then applied and the patient left comfortable. The equipment is cleared away. If there is profuse discharge, it may be easier to clean the vulva by pouring lotion from a jug over the area and then drying carefully. This is usually called jug douching or swabbing. It is necessary to sit the patient on a bedpan to receive the lotion before carrying out this procedure.

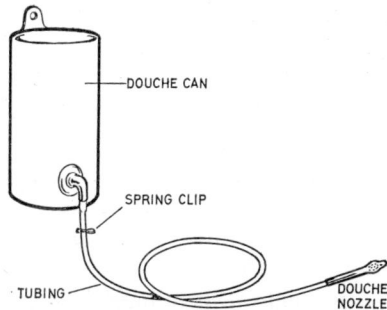

Fig. 43.—Apparatus for a Vaginal Douche.

DOUCHE CAN

SPRING CLIP

TUBING

DOUCHE NOZZLE

Vaginal douching.—The vagina is a hollow tube which may need irrigation before surgery, or if the patient has a pessary in position, the apparatus required includes a douche can, tubing and a catheter or a douche nozzle which may be glass or plastic.

This is usually a sterile procedure but is often carried out by women in their own homes. The lotions used are similar to those for vulval swabbing, and are prepared at body temperature. The patient should be allowed to pass urine, and then be sat on a clean bedpan. Air is expelled from the apparatus, the vulva is swabbed and the nozzle introduced approximately 5 cms. into the vagina. The fluid is allowed to flow freely, and will return into the bedpan: 600–1200 mls. of fluid are used. When the douche is finished, the area is dried thoroughly and a vulval pad is applied if necessary.

COMPLICATIONS FOLLOWING OPERATION

Several complications may follow surgery, due either to the operation itself, or to the anaesthetic. They may be avoided, or minimised in many cases, by careful pre- and post-operative care. Any persistent symptoms should be reported to the ward sister or doctor.

Vomiting.—This is a distressing occurrence for the patient and will cause pain if there is an abdominal wound. It may be due to inadequate preparation, the anaesthetic itself, or to too liberal administration of fluids in the immediate post-operative period. Another reason may be fear, and it should be remembered that many people are very suggestible and the vomit bowl should not be too conspicuous. Persistent vomiting continuing 24 hours after the operation is a more serious symptom which may need prolonged treatment. Mild vomiting may be relieved by attending to the patient's general comfort—i.e. offering a bedpan or urinal if necessary, changing the patient's position and giving the appropriate analgesic and allowing the patient to rest; a mouthwash will be refreshing and fluids should be restricted.

Some anti-emetic drug, e.g. chlorpromazine (Largactil) may be prescribed.

Hiccoughs.—This may follow surgery at the upper abdomen —that is, on those organs near the diaphragm. It is also distressing and causes pain. Sips of water may help and sedatives may be necessary; inhalations of oxygen (95%) and carbon dioxide (5%) are sometimes given.

Chest complications.—Following surgery or a general anaesthetic, the patient may have difficulty in breathing: this may be due to the site of operation, the anaesthetic or simply that the patient is confined to bed. Deep-breathing exercises should be encouraged before and after surgery, and the patient's position changed regularly if he is unable to do this for himself. Early signs of chest complications are a cough and a raised respiration rate, and later a rise in temperature. Treatment is as described above and as ordered by the doctor.

Retention of urine.—Difficulty in passing urine is common, particularly after low abdominal or pelvic surgery. It may be due to pain, apprehension, inadequate fluid intake or simply to handling of the bladder or associated structures at operation. Since many people have difficulty in using a bedpan, one way of overcoming this is to help the patient into a more normal position: in men, this is achieved by letting them sit on the edge of the bed—in women, by assisting them to a commode at the bedside. Fluids by mouth will help, provided the bladder is not already distended, and simple medicines such as mist. potassium citrate (mild diuretic) may be given. If the patient has not passed urine within a few hours of operation, the ward sister should be informed, as it may be necessary to pass a catheter. Although catheterisation should be avoided if possible, it is a mistake to "wait and see" beyond a certain point, as a distended bladder causes considerable pain and distress to the patient.

The drug carbachol, which contracts the plain muscle of the bladder, may be prescribed.

In many instances, patients who undergo surgery of the lower abdomen or pelvis, return from theatre with a self-retaining catheter in position, and this is left in position for 48 to 72 hours.

Venous thrombosis.—This has already been described in some detail (page 58), and it is the result of lack of movement in a patient confined to bed. Treatment will be ordered by the doctor, and consists of a course of anticoagulant drugs to prevent further clot formation. The term phlebitis is used to describe the inflammatory condition, but thrombophlebitis is the more common term, since clot formation is usual when a vein is inflamed.

Wound infection.—Unfortunately, this is a common postoperative complication. Measures to prevent cross-infection have already been described (page 109); as far as the wound is concerned, the use of strict aseptic techniques in the theatre and ward will do much to lessen the risk, but sometimes the source of infection is the patient himself—e.g. his nose, throat or skin.

Wound infection shows itself in many ways: locally, the nurse may observe reddening of the skin, obvious pus formation or failure of healing. Generally, the patient will feel less well, may complain of pain, and a rise in his temperature, pulse, and respiration rates will be noted. Treatment is as prescribed and will depend on the causative organism and the symptoms exhibited. The organisms causing concern at present are staphylococcus aureus, E. Coli and Proteus.

Shock.—Shock is the term used to describe a state of circulatory collapse, and occurs to some degree following any injury or operation. It is characterised by pallor, sweating, a rapid, feeble pulse, low blood pressure and shallow respirations. The degree of shock can be minimised by careful preparation and after-care. It is aggravated by pain, fear, loss of body fluid and deep or prolonged anaesthesia, and can therefore be lessened by relieving pain after operation, reassurance and explanation before and after surgery, and the use of intravenous fluids where necessary.

Many patients returning from theatre exhibit symptoms of shock, but with normal care these quickly disappear. Observations are made, as previously described, and any unusual symptoms reported and treated. The use of additional warmth is not encouraged in most cases, since it can have the effect of making the patient sweat, so losing more body fluid and aggravating the condition.

Haemorrhage.—As a post-operative complication, severe bleeding is not common: it is sometimes seen following such operations as adeno-tonsillectomy, where it may be difficult for the surgeon to tie off the cut vessels. If haemorrhage occurs, it is either external or internal. If external, the blood is seen, the condition reported, diagnosed and treated quickly; if internal, the usual observations will lead to the diagnosis, since the signs and symptoms are a rapid, rising pulse rate, restlessness, pallor, sweating and increased respiration rate. The treatment will be ordered by the surgeon and may involve blood transfusion and the return of the patient to theatre.

Paralytic ileus.—As a result of excessive handling of the gut during surgery, or sometimes due to infection before operation, e.g. following a perforated appendix, a paralysis of the small intestine develops. This is a serious condition characterised by persistent severe vomiting leading to dehydration and collapse, shock and absence of bowel sounds. The basic nursing care is that of any seriously ill patient: treatment will include stopping all food and fluids by mouth and keeping the stomach empty by means of suction applied to a naso-gastric tube: fluids will be given by an alternative route, e.g. intravenously, and this regimen continued until bowel sounds return, which is a sign that peristaltic movements are present once more.

Chapter XIII

THE YOUNG AND THE OLD IN HOSPITAL

Among the patients admitted to hospital, certain groups present problems related to their age as well as to their conditions. In the young these problems arise as full independence has not been achieved, whereas for the elderly the problem is to accept increasing dependence on others as their health fails.

THE CHILD IN HOSPITAL

The ward.—Whenever possible, children should be nursed in a separate ward or hospital which caters for their needs. Cubicles are normally provided for the very young and in many instances accommodation is provided for the mother. This is especially important for the "toddler", as at this age the child is very dependent on her and likely to suffer emotionally if prolonged separation occurs. Visiting hours should be flexible and mothers encouraged to carry out the routine care of their own children as they would at home: e.g. bathing and feeding.

A children's ward is frequently untidy and often noiser than an adult ward. Visitors come and go at all times during the day and the atmosphere is more informal. Part of the nurses' routine duties will be to play with and amuse the children—this is made much easier if a separate "play" or day room is available, since most of them will be up for part of the day.

Two problems are the prevention of cross-infection and accidents. It is difficult to prevent infection spreading since children are naturally gregarious and exchange toys and sweets. Accidents can be avoided by keeping cupboards locked, by seeing that cot sides are securely fastened and by removing obvious hazards. Restrainers may be used to keep a child in his cot, but allow him freedom to play.

Admission.—The admission of a child is similar to that previously described; details are normally obtained from his parents and must include whether or not he has been baptised —and if not, his parents' wishes in an emergency, details of vaccination and immunisation, and the infectious diseases the child has had. With the baby and toddler, it is necessary to obtain details of how and when he is fed, his toilet habits and his vocabulary.

The mother should be allowed to undress the child and stay with him for a while. A favourite toy or plaything will provide a link with home and often helps to comfort him when his parents leave. Before they go the nurse must make sure that an operation consent form has been signed and should explain

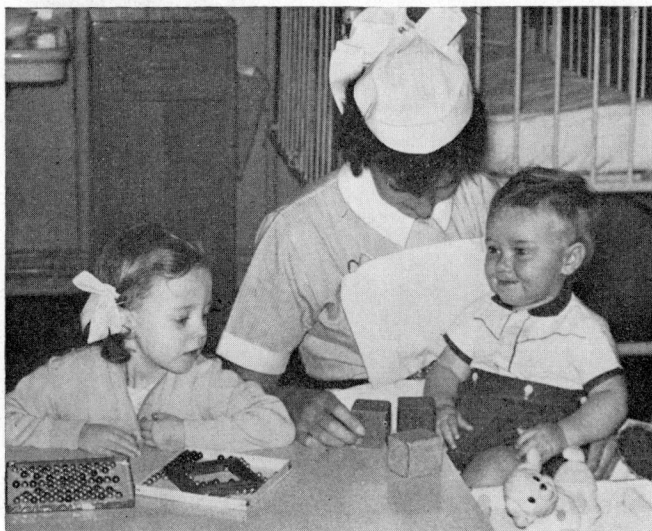

FIG. 44.—"Part of the nurse's routine duties."

any ward rules with regard to food or sweets brought in by visitors. The young child is likely to cry when his parents go, in fact this is a normal reaction. The older child will soon accept a new routine, provided his parents visit regularly and that truthful answers and explanations are given in reply to questions.

Bathing a baby.—Before the baby is undressed, the necessary toilet articles and clean clothes are collected and placed within easy reach of the bath. Draughts are excluded and the bath prepared with water which is comfortably warm to the nurse's elbow. It is advisable for her to wear a rubber apron, and a gown and mask may be worn. A low chair is placed by the bath and the nurse sits down with the baby on her lap; she undresses him, leaving his nappy in place, and wraps him in a large towel.

189

His face is washed, using clean water and cotton wool swabs, and dried, using a soft towel; as a rule it is unnecessary to clean inside his nose, ears or mouth. To wash his hair, the nurse holds him under her left arm with the hand and wrist supporting his head—his hair is then washed and dried.

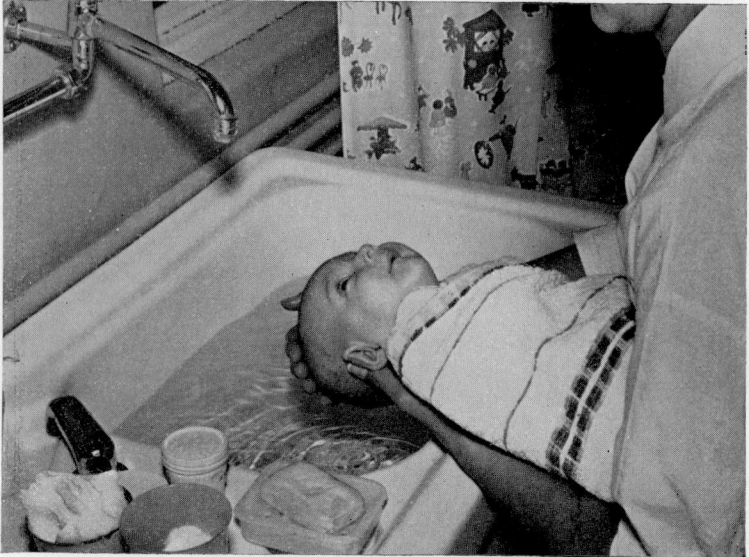

FIG. 45.—Washing a Baby's Hair.

With the baby on her knee, the nurse loosens the towel, removes the nappy and soaps his body all over; she lifts him into the bath to rinse off the soap and allows him to kick for a few minutes—his head must be supported as before. He is lifted out of the bath and carefully dried, special attention being paid to the creases and folds in his skin; a light dusting of talcum powder can be applied and he is then dressed. The time of day when a baby is bathed is immaterial, but it should be before rather than after a feed.

The toddler is usually bathed in the bathroom; it is important to remember that he is in a strange place, and used to a different routine. It may help if a familiar toy is available and the nurse should not attempt to hurry him.

Older children are bathed in the same way as adults.

Feeding infants and children.—If a baby is being breast fed, his mother will be admitted with him; if he is bottle fed, the nurse will obtain details of his feed from her. Unless contra-indicated, the baby continues with his usual type and amount of feed.

The majority of bottle-fed babies in this country have some form of dried milk. Instructions for preparing the feeds are given on the tin and should be carefully followed. In general, a

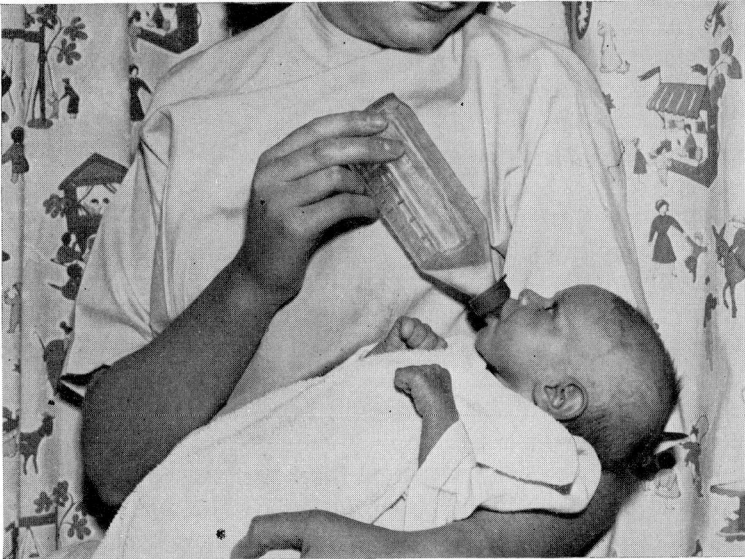

FIG. 46.—"Milk—not air."

baby requires 75–90 mls. of fluid per pound of his body weight in 24 hours.

For example: a 3·6 Kgs. baby needs 600–720 mls. per day, which can be given as 5 feeds of 120–150 mls.; it is customary to omit the 2 a.m. feed.

Other types of milk are evaporated milk—again instructions are given on the tin—and ordinary milk, which must be boiled, sweetened and diluted according to the baby's age. The amounts of fluid are as mentioned earlier.

Care of the bottles and teats is important as stale milk is an ideal breeding ground for bacteria. They should be cleaned

191

thoroughly after each feed and can then either be boiled for five minutes, or stored in hypochlorite solution (Milton).

Cod liver oil and orange or blackcurrant juice should be given to bottle-fed babies from the age of 3 to 4 weeks.

The baby should be changed before being fed and the feed warmed by standing the bottle in a jug of hot water. The nurse washes her hands, puts on a gown and perhaps a mask and sits comfortably on a chair with the baby on her lap. His gown is protected by a feeder, the cover removed from the teat and the temperature of the feed tested by allowing a few drops of milk to fall on the nurse's forearm. The hole in the teat should be big enough to let the milk drip through at a steady rate when the bottle is inverted. During the feed, the baby's head must be supported and the bottle held so that the baby sucks milk and not air.

Half-way through the feed, the bottle is removed and the baby's wind brought up by holding him in an upright position and rubbing or patting his back. The rest of the feed is then given and his wind brought up again. If necessary, his nappy is changed again, and he is put back in his cot, lying on his side; most babies sleep after a feed.

From the age of 3 to 6 months, solid foods are introduced and are given with a teaspoon before the bottle feed. By 9 to 12 months the baby will try to hold the spoon and will then begin to feed himself. Although it is quicker for the nurse to feed a toddler, he should be encouraged to help himself as much as possible, suitable protection being provided for the child, the nurse and the floor.

If an older child is on complete rest, he is fed in the same way as an adult.

Observations.—The observations to be made in the case of an ill child are similar to those already described. However a child's condition can alter much more rapidly than an adult's and in certain cases treatment is needed more urgently; for example, young children with diarrhoea and vomiting become shocked and dehydrated very quickly, and an upper respiratory tract infection can prove fatal in a few hours, if untreated. Careful observation is therefore of extreme importance, even more so when the child is too young to communicate.

Examination and treatment.—When the young child is examined by the doctor, or if unpleasant procedures are to be carried out, it is usually much easier for everyone if the mother can be present to reassure and hold him. If this is not possible, a nurse with whom the child has established a good relationship should assist the doctor.

When an injection or similar treatment is to be given, it is kinder for a second nurse to hold the child even if he appears to be co-operative, so that the procedure is over as quickly as possible.

For the older child, a simple explanation is all that is necessary and most children are perfectly reasonable and co-operate well if approached sensibly.

Medicines and drugs.—The dosage of drugs varies with the size and age of the child. Two simple formulae will give the nurse an idea of how to work out a dose, if the amount needed for an adult is known.

Young's rule. $\dfrac{\text{Age of child}}{\text{Age} + 12} \times \text{Adult dose} = \text{Child's dose}.$

e.g. A 4-year-old is to be given Nembutal.

$\dfrac{4}{4 + 12} \times 180$ mgms.

$\dfrac{1}{4} \times 180$ mgms. $= 45$ mgms.

A more accurate method is by weight.

Clark's rule. $\dfrac{\text{Weight of child in pounds}}{150} \times \text{Adult dose}$

$= \text{Child's dose}$

e.g. A 15-lb. baby is to have chloral hydrate.

$\dfrac{15}{150} \times 1.5$ Gms.

$\dfrac{1}{10} \times 1.5$ G. $= 150$ mgms.

As well as this, it must be remembered that tolerance to certain drugs is different. For example, small children have a poor tolerance of morphine and it is not often used; but atropine is tolerated very well and an adult dose is often given to quite young children.

Many medicines are dispensed in a pleasant syrup mixture, and it is usual to give a sweet after medicine has been taken. Penicillin is used as an oral mixture to a larger extent than with adults; this avoids the use of repeated injections.

Aids to diagnosis and treatment.—Many of the procedures already described (Chapter X) are used in paediatric wards. The difference lies in the approach to the child, the size of the equipment and a wider use of general as distinct from local anaesthetics when endoscopy is performed.

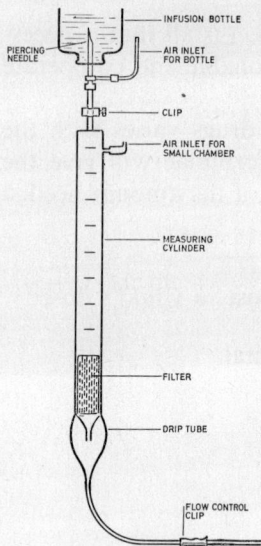

FIG. 47.—Intravenous Set for Infants.

Intravenous fluids.—Because a baby is small, the amounts of fluid given intravenously are also small; the total amount of circulating blood in a newborn baby is only 400 to 500 mls., whereas the average adult has 4 to 5 litres. The baby is not able to cope with sudden changes in the amount or composition of circulating fluid; this means that great care is necessary both in estimating the amount to be given and in seeing that it is not exceeded. To help in this, special intravenous infusion sets are used which incorporate a small chamber—30 to 100 mls.; this is filled at intervals from the main container and the infusion supplied directly from the small cylinder; it is therefore impossible for more than 30 to 100 mls. to be given until the small cylinder is re-filled.

The needles used are small, and because the veins are smaller and more difficult to puncture, the technique of cutting down and the use of polythene tubing is more common than in adults. The veins of the scalp are sometimes used.

Pre- and post-operative care.—Basically this is the same as for an adult; the older child must be given a simple explanation of what is to happen—and if, for example, he is having his tonsils out, he should be warned that his throat will be sore afterwards.

The period of starvation before an anaesthetic may be shorter, since the child's blood sugar falls more quickly. It is best for him if he is asleep when he arrives in the theatre, and pre-medication is given with this in mind. After operation, many anaesthetists like to keep the child in the anaesthetic room until he is conscious, or at least able to cough and swallow.

The nursing care is as already described following operation, and the post-operative period is usually uneventful. The dangers of being confined to bed are less, since most children are active soon after operation. The child who lies quietly in bed for hours, taking little interest in his surroundings, is either very ill or emotionally disturbed.

THE ELDERLY IN HOSPITAL

It is difficult to define old age; some people are old at 65, others remarkably young at 80. When an old person becomes ill, it is usual for him to be admitted to one of the general wards of his local hospital; his subsequent care depends on what is wrong with him, but as in many cases prolonged treatment is necessary, it may be decided to transfer him to a geriatric ward —that is, a ward for old people.

Children and grandchildren nowadays find it increasingly difficult to care for their elderly sick relatives, partly due to smaller houses and flats and partly to the fact that both husband and wife go out to work and are unable to provide the continuous care necessary. For these reasons, difficulties arise for old people when the time comes for them to go home; equally, some are admitted to geriatric wards simply because they cannot care for themselves any longer, even though not acutely ill.

In recent years the approach to the geriatric patient has altered considerably and emphasis is now placed on rehabilitation, so that wherever possible he is able to resume an active useful life. Many geriatric wards in general hospitals are quite unsuitable for those patients who require a home and supervision rather than detailed nursing care. For this reason, many authorities provide "half-way" houses to which the convalescent patient can go to be assessed as regards his subsequent discharge or transfer to an old people's home.

The geriatric ward.—Ideally the equipment in a geriatric ward should be designed with the elderly in mind. Beds need to be lower than is usual in hospital, since many old people have considerable difficulty in getting in or out. Floors should not be highly polished since some patients will be unsteady on their feet and all furniture should be adapted to suit the needs of the patient—for example, the baths should be low, have some type of handrail and if necessary a wooden fitting can be added to provide a seat.

General care.—All nurses in training will nurse elderly patients, whether the training school has separate geriatric wards or not. The principles involved in their care are the same as for any other patient, but certain details must be emphasised because of the patient's age and decline in activity.

With advancing years, the skin becomes less elastic and the subcutaneous tissues less well nourished. It is unfortunate that many old people develop bed sores rapidly when admitted to hospital. Two reasons may be a change in their habits, or an alteration in their food and fluid intake. Very little research has been undertaken until recently with regard to the best method of preventing pressure sores, but reports now indicate that frequent moving (2-hourly) and attention to fluid intake and diet are far more effective than the traditional methods of massage and local applications.

Incontinence has been thought to be inevitable in many elderly patients, but this is not necessarily true and can be avoided in many cases. The use of commodes and toilet chairs has helped and these and bedpans and urinals must be offered at frequent intervals. Many old people are afraid to drink, because they fear that if they do the result will be a wet bed; the nurse can overcome this fear by explaining that there is always someone available to help them to the toilet or fetch a bedpan. If the patient is incontinent, the use of disposable absorbent pads, placed under the buttocks, will minimise the amount of wet and soiled linen.

Old people, like children, are very susceptible to sudden changes in temperature; this should be remembered when considering the comfort of the patient—whether he is lying in bed, sitting in a chair or being taken to the bath. Extra blankets, shawls, bed jackets and bed socks can be used and will be much appreciated.

196

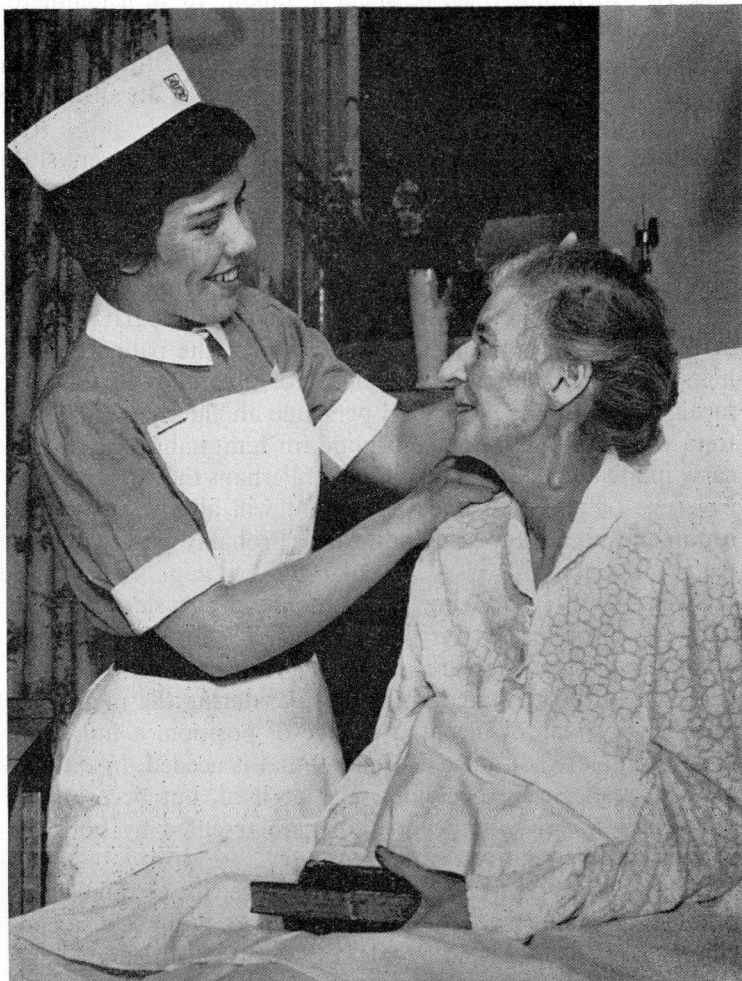

FIG. 48.—". . . can be very rewarding."
(*By kind permission of the United Sheffield Hospitals*).

Cheerfulness, patience and understanding are invaluable qualities in any nurse, but are essential when caring for the elderly. Much time must be spent in talking to, or listening to, the patient. As with a small child, it is often quicker to do things for the patient than to help him to do them himself, but as soon as he is well enough he must be encouraged to do all that he can even if this is time-consuming.

Meals.—The calorie needs of old people are fewer, since metabolism is slower and activity less. In addition, many elderly people wear dentures which are not always comfortable or a good fit. If this is so, they will find it difficult to eat any but the softest foods. Consideration must therefore be given to ordering suitable foods which are nutritious, palatable and at the same time present no difficulties for the patient. Small helpings should be given and plenty of time allowed for each meal; it is pointless to try and persuade an elderly patient that food which he does not like is good for him; habits are formed early in life and are difficult to break. Perhaps the most popular beverage of all is tea and the patient will always be grateful for an unexpected cup, as at home he is probably used to making tea at all hours.

Sleep.—With advancing years the need for sleep lessens; many old people sleep very lightly and only for short periods. Sometimes, when they are admitted to hospital, they become restless and disorientated if they awake during the night. The offer of a bedpan or urinal, a change of position, a hot drink and above all reassurance is often all that is needed. In extreme cases of restlessness, bed-sides may be used, but occasionally they make the situation worse and are resented by both the patient and his relatives.

Drugs.—With increasing age, tolerance to certain drugs becomes less and smaller doses are required. Some, e.g. scopolamine, seem to make old people restless and disorientated and for this reason are not commonly used.

Social problems.—When an old person is admitted to hospital, many problems arise which need prompt attention since they affect the patient's peace of mind and so hinder recovery. These problems include the care of their husband/wife and home, and such practical details as who will collect the old age pension and attend to pets or other commitments. For those who live alone there is always the fear that incapacity may prevent a return home. These and other worries are referred to the medical social worker, who will be able to help. If the patient is nursed in a general ward, visiting time may be upsetting as many old people have few friends or relatives who are able or willing to visit.

It is difficult to generalise about the care of old people in hospital, since the reasons for admission and the aims of treatment are so varied; as mentioned, some are in hospital because they are acutely ill and so need intensive nursing care, others for social reasons who simply need a home, general care and in some cases rehabilitation.

Difficulties also arise since some are nursed in general wards of the hospital and others in geriatric units, where the approach and pace are different.

Although caring for old people is undramatic and heavy, it can be rewarding for the nurse and provides an opportunity to practice basic nursing skills rarely found elsewhere.

Chapter XIV

DISCHARGE FROM HOSPITAL

Many patients leaving hospital need a period of convalescence before they are able to resume their normal occupation. If a patient is unable to arrange this for himself, or if supervision is still necessary, the medical social worker may be able to make arrangements for him to go to a convalescent home; in these cases the cost is borne by the National Health Service. Before the patient leaves hospital it is important that he fully understands any instructions given him by the doctor and is proficient in any treatment that he is to carry on at home, e.g. the administration of insulin, or the care of a colostomy. When dietary restrictions are necessary, it is essential that the diet sheets issued are practical, simple to follow and that the cost of the foods mentiond are within the patient's means. It is helpful if the person who normally does the family cooking is seen by the dietitian, or ward sister. Occasionally the doctor prescribes medicines for the patient to take home with him; these are obtained from the pharmacy in the usual way and are dispensed in correctly labelled containers. If the patient is to attend a follow-up clinic in the out-patient department, an appointment is made for him and a card issued giving the date and time when he is to be seen.

Medical certificates will have been given at intervals during his stay in hospital so that sickness benefit can be obtained; on discharge, any further certificates needed will be obtained from his general practitioner.

Any items belonging to the patient which have been stored by the hospital during his stay are returned to him and his signature obtained for them. The time of discharge from the ward is arranged in advance with his relatives, who bring the necessary clothes and usually arrange some form of transport. In certain circumstances an ambulance may be ordered.

Rarely, a patient wishes to take his own discharge against medical advice; if he cannot be dissuaded from this course of action, the risks are explained to him and he must sign the appropriate form to this effect.

The empty bed is stripped and all linen and blankets sent to the laundry; the bed frame and locker are washed with soap and water. When these are dry, and the mattress and pillows aired, the bed is remade, using clean linen, ready for the next patient. All charts, notes and X-rays are collected together and sent to the records department. It is usual for the doctor to write to the general practitioner advising him of the patient's discharge, the treatment carried out in hospital and details of any further care necessary. This further care may have been arranged in advance but will be supervised by the general practitioner. The services available to the patient at home are those provided by the local health authority.

LOCAL HEALTH AUTHORITY SERVICES

District nurses.   Ambulances.
District midwives.   Care and after-care services.
Health visitors.   Maternity and child welfare clinics.
Home helps.   Vaccination and immunisation.
              Health centres—in some areas.

District nurses are State Registered Nurses who may also be State Certified Midwives and who have in many cases undergone further training to introduce them to the problems of nursing patients in their own homes. As a rule they are provided with some form of transport since the area they cover is large. It is becoming common for State Enrolled Nurses to work alongside district nurses.

The increased pressure on hospital beds has meant that many patients have to wait for a long period before being admitted to hospital, while others are being discharged from hospital earlier than in the past; this has increased the amount of care and supervision necessary at home which is carried out by the district nurse. Patients are referred to her either by the local hospital or by general practitioners with whom she works closely. Among her problems are the age range of her patients and the wide variation in the scope of her duties. These will include general care and toilet of those confined to bed, injections of various drugs including insulin, dressings, and in fact any nursing treatments which may be needed. She has to plan her day so that those patients needing prompt attention are seen early, while those for whom her visit may be the only contact of the day may have her unhurried attention. The size of her district varies considerably, according to whether it is in a crowded town or a rural community. In both cases relief nurses are provided to ensure a continuous service when she is off duty. Many authorities employ male State Registered Nurses to care for men who are sick at home.

District midwives.—A district midwife is normally a State Registered Nurse who has undertaken further training to become a State Certified Midwife and has chosen to work in the local health authority service rather than the hospital service.

Her duties are more specific than those of the district nurse, and are concerned with the care of women during pregnancy, the delivery of babies born at home and the care of the mother and child for the first 14 days after birth. She works with either the general practitioner concerned or the doctor at the local maternity and child welfare clinic, but she may be entirely responsible for the delivery of the baby. Should unforeseen complications arise during labour, she can call on an emergency service provided by the nearest maternity unit. Owing to the present acute shortage of maternity beds in hospital, the district midwife may also care for those women who have had their babies in hospital, but have been discharged home within the first 14 days.

Health visitors.—The health visitor is a State Registered Nurse with further post-graduate experience which includes midwifery and a 9-month course to obtain the Health Visitors' Certificate awarded by the Royal Society for the Promotion of Health. Her work is concerned more with the social aspects of disease and its prevention than with the detailed bedside care carried out by the district nurse.

She takes over from the district midwife at the end of the 14-day period following the birth of a baby, and follows the fortunes and misfortunes of the child throughout the pre-school years, both at home and at the local maternity and child welfare clinic. She may also be the school nurse, in which case she will see him at intervals throughout his school career. The health visitor is a welcome guest in many homes, but she has no right of entry and therefore her success depends on her approach and personality. Her work lies more with those families who find the problems of life difficult than with those who are well able to cope.

Much of her time is also spent with the elderly people in her district and it is her duty to see that they take advantage of all the services available to them, such as "Meals on Wheels", chiropody service and similar facilities. Lonely old people may be brought to her notice by doctors, neighbours, friends or relatives and should she find that the old person needs nursing attention she can contact the district nurse. In country districts she may in fact also be the district nurse and district midwife.

Home helps.—It is not a statutory duty of the local health authority to provide a home help service, but in fact many do. The qualifications necessary for the women who provide this service are tact, a pleasant manner and the ability to run a home. Because of this many home helps are housewives undertaking part-time work. They are paid at a fixed rate by the local authority who recover part or all of the money from those to whom the service is given, depending on their ability to pay.

The service is provided mainly as a temporary measure in cases where the housewife is sick and unable to care for her home and family, and for women following childbirth, and as a permanent service for the elderly and disabled in their own homes. The frequency of the service varies with the need—being daily to undertake all housework in some cases, or weekly to do the shopping and heavy chores in others.

The home help service is in no way a nursing service, and unfortunately, at present, the demand is far greater than the supply.

Ambulances.—The ambulance service is best known to the general public for its response to emergencies; but these only form a part of the work. Ambulance stations may be located at one hospital, but their vehicles serve a large area which includes several hospitals. The day-to-day work will include fetching people from their homes to attend clinics or have some form of treatment, if they are unable or unfit to use public transport; taking home patients who have been in hospital and are unable to make other arrangements; and occasionally transporting a patient who is being transferred from one hospital to another. When ambulances are required for hospital patients, the ward sister or medical social worker makes arrangements with the transport officer; outside hospital they can only be obtained by a general practitioner, or through the "999 emergency" service. The drivers and attendants are trained in first aid.

Care and after-care.—The local health authority is empowered to provide help to those persons suffering from such conditions as tuberculosis and mental illness. This is not a medical service and aims at rehabilitating the patient by using existing voluntary and statutory services, for example—home helps, the disablement resettlement officer and the Women's Royal Voluntary Service.

Psychiatric social workers are now employed by many authorities to help those patients attending hospital as out-patients of the psychiatric clinics.

Maternity and child welfare clinics.—These clinics have already been mentioned in connection with the work of the district midwife and health visitor. The young mother is advised to take her baby to the local clinic at regular intervals, so that his development and progress can be observed and advice given regarding feeding and any other problems. The clinic does not provide a service for the ill child and if any disease or abnormality is found, he is referred to his general practitioner or local hospital.

At the clinic the baby is weighed and examined by the medical officer of health or one of his assistants; subsidised foods may be obtained and vaccination and immunisation are available. Sessions for different age groups are often held on different days, and normally the frequency of the visits becomes less as the child grows older. Some of the work at the clinics is carried out by voluntary helpers, particularly members of the Women's Royal Voluntary Service.

Vaccination and immunisation.—Research into communicable diseases has led to the development of many vaccines which protect the individual from specific infections for varying lengths of time. In general it is thought advisable to have children immunised at an early age and programmes are arranged by each local authority to protect the children in their area. These plans aim to reduce the number of injections to a minimum and to give maximum protection at the age when it is most likely to be required. The programme usually starts at between 3 to 6 months of age and continues over the following 12 to 18 months; "booster" doses are given just before the child starts school and in some cases when he is older. These programmes are available to all, but there is no compulsion; details are explained by the staff at the clinic, or by the general practitioner, either of whom may carry out the programme. At present protection is offered against the following diseases:

Diphtheria.	Poliomyelitis.
Whooping cough.	Smallpox.
Tetanus.	Tuberculosis.
Measles.	

Health centres.—When the National Health Service came into being it was envisaged that many of the local authority services could be combined with general practitioner surgeries and other services such as X-rays, dental clinics and chiropody in the same building—the Health centre. For the first 20 years of the N.H.S. few were built, but in 1968 and 1969 over 100 were opened or were in process of building. The next few years should see a great increase in the number of Health centres and group practice clinics.

Other services available.—Many services have been instituted by voluntary organisations which are used and in some cases subsidised by the local authority. Examples are the "Meals on Wheels" service, started by the Women's Royal Voluntary Service, which provides a hot meal 2 or 3 times a week for those in need, and the Red Cross and St. John's organisations, who provide various accessories needed for patients confined to bed at home; these accessories include backrests, bedpans and urinals and waterproof sheeting.

CARE OF THE DYING

Not all patients recover from their illness and some die in hospital. Occasionally death is sudden and unexpected, but in many cases the patient will have been critically ill for some time. For the majority of nurses in training, this will be their first experience of death, and many are understandably apprehensive and uncertain of their own ability to cope with the situation and help the relatives.

The basic nursing care of the dying patient is concerned primarily with his comfort and the relief of any distressing symptoms. The care of the mouth is important since it may become very dry, owing to the limited food and fluid intake; if the patient is unconscious or semi-conscious, the eyes may need frequent attention, and in the terminal stages he may be incontinent.

Many ward sisters prefer to nurse a very ill, or dying patient in a side ward, which is less distressing for the other patients and a help to the relatives. Otherwise, the bed is usually moved to a corner of the ward and the bed curtains kept drawn. It is usual for the relatives to be allowed to visit at any time and if they, or the patient himself, wish to see the priest or minister, this should be arranged immediately. Different denominations and religions have different customs and rites connected with dying, and the nurse should make sure that she is familiar with those applicable to her patients. She will find that her own faith is a great help at these times—not only to herself, but to the patient and his relatives.

If relatives wish to stay with the patient for long periods, the nurse should see that they do not become over tired and should encourage them to go out for a short while at intervals. During the night they can often rest in a room provided away from the ward.

When death occurs it must be certified by the doctor or sister in charge and the relatives told. After seeing the patient they may be offered a cup of tea, and arrangements made for them to go home. They should be asked to return to the hospital the next day, to collect any clothing and other belongings, and the death certificate.

Notices of death are sent to various departments, including the Central Nursing Office.

LAST OFFICES

The body is laid flat and the top bedclothes removed, leaving only a sheet; the limbs are straightened and the eyes closed—it may be necessary to place damp wool swabs on the eyelids to keep them closed. A bandage is placed under the jaw and tied round the top of the head to keep the mouth shut: any apparatus—e.g. I.V. infusion—is disconnected and any naso-gastric or urinary drainage tubes are removed. After this the body is covered with the sheet and left for a period of time. The nurse empties the locker and lists the items in the appropriate book;

these will be collected and signed for by the relatives next day.

Two nurses prepare a trolley similar to that required for a blanket bath, with the addition of a shroud and mortuary sheet, labels and needles and cotton. At the bedside, a fresh dressing is applied to any wound, if necessary covering this with waterproof strapping. Local practice should be followed with regard to drainage tubes which may be left in place. The body is washed, the nails, hair and mouth attended to—dentures which have been removed should be replaced—and a light plug of wool inserted into the rectum. The body is dressed in the shroud and labels attached to identify it—one is commonly stitched on to the front of the shroud. The details on the label should include the name, age, ward, religion and date and time of death. All jewellery is removed, except in the case of the wedding ring which is often impossible to remove, and in any case the relatives' wishes should be ascertained about this.

Many nurses find that this procedure is less disturbing than they had imagined and look on it as a last service rendered to the patient.

The body is placed on the mortuary sheet which is wrapped round it to make a complete covering; a further label may be placed on the outside of the sheet. When the body is ready, a trolley is brought to the ward and in some cases a nurse will accompany it to the mortuary or chapel.

All linen is sent to the laundry, and the bed and locker washed.

Should no relatives be present, it is the responsibility of the hospital to notify them immediately and to put into safe keeping any valuables belonging to the patient until such time as they can be collected.

Chapter XV

THE NURSE IN TRAINING

RESIDENCE

In some instances the nurse is expected to live in for at least the
first year of her training. This is a reasonable condition, since in
many cases she will have chosen a hospital some way away from
home and, after the Introductory Course, will be working
irregular hours and going on night duty. For some, the restrictions of the nurses' home will seem tedious, but the rules are
only those necessary for a happy community in which members
share the amenities. In fact the regulations in many nurses'
homes are far less strict than in some women's university hos-
tels, and are basically simply a combination of consideration
for others and good manners.

The person in charge may be a senior member of the nursing
staff—the home sister—or a non-nursing warden. In either case
she is responsible for the smooth running of the home and in
some cases is also in charge of the nurses' clinic or sick bay. It
is usual for a clinic to be held daily, to which nurses report if
they are not well; the doctor in charge may be a member of the
hospital medical staff, or a local general practitioner who comes
in to see sick staff. In some teaching hospitals, the nurses' health
is supervised by the university student health service. Except in
an emergency, it is important to report sick at the stated times
as most people do at a doctor's surgery; however, there is
always someone to whom a nurse can report if she suddenly
feels ill. If she is told to remain off duty for more than three
days, then a medical certificate must be obtained for insurance
purposes.

In some hospitals, nurses are asked to sign in when returning
late, or after sleeping out; the object of this is to ensure that,
in an emergency, all staff can be accounted for. When going on
holiday it is customary to leave a forwarding address for post
and to write to the Senior Nursing Officer and/or home sister
a few days before returning.

Many nurses choose to live out when this is allowed and they
can find suitable accommodation. Obviously, if a nurse's

parents live near the hospital, she may choose to live at home. Reasonable accommodation may be difficult to find at a moderate rent, and often it is necessary for several nurses to share rooms or a flat; this is an excellent arrangement as far as sharing expenses and "chores" are concerned, but may have disadvantages if some are on night duty and the others on day duty.

Although it is possible for a non-resident nurse to be seen at the nurses' clinic if she is taken ill on duty, she should find a general practitioner near her flat who will accept her on his list.

TRAINING ALLOWANCE AND CONDITIONS OF SERVICE

A nurse in training is paid an allowance which increases slightly each year; from this deductions are made towards the cost of uniform, laundry and accommodation if resident. On joining the Health Service she is automatically included in the National Health Service superannuation scheme to which both she and her employer pay monthly contributions; if she leaves the Health Service, her contributions—less tax—are repayed; otherwise they accumulate towards her pension. She also pays income tax, national insurance and state pension contributions. Meals are paid for when they are taken.

Paid sick leave is allowed according to her length of service, but if she has sick leave in excess of 7 days for each year of training, the date at which she can take her Final Examinations may be affected.

Holidays are given as follows: 4 weeks in each of the first 2 years of training and 5 weeks in the third year.

These allowances and conditions of service are laid down by the Nurses and Midwives Whitley Council. This body has a management side representing the employers—Board of Governors and Regional Hospital Boards—and a staff side, representing all grades of nursing and midwifery staff; the two sides negotiate all salaries and conditions of service. The staff side is made up of representatives of all large professional organisations and trades unions with nurse members.

PROFESSIONAL ORGANISATIONS

The Royal College of Nursing was formed in 1916 and received its Royal Charter in 1939. It has recently become amalgamated with the National Council of Nurses, to become the largest single organisation for trained nurses in this country, and the national representative on the International Council of Nurses.

Its aims include the maintenance of professional standards and the promotion of the science and art of nursing, and it also organises many post-registration courses in nurse education and administration. By virtue of its size, the Royal College of Nursing is in a strong position to put forward the views and aims of the nursing profession, and it also supports individual members who need legal advice or representation.

The Student Nurses' Association, to which the nurse in training may belong, is part of the Royal College of Nursing; its aims are similar to those of the College, and through its association with the National Union of Students it provides many amenities, including discount on various goods and facilities for holidays at reduced rates. Members may also take advantage of hostel accommodation in London. The Student Nurses' Association has a Central Representative Council, whose members are student nurses, elected by their colleagues, from all over the country. Members may make use of the library facilities at the Royal College of Nursing—either directly or by post. Each year a speech-making contest is held, starting with area competitions and culminating in a final contest in London.

When members of the Student Nurses' Association become State Registered, they are able to join the Royal College of Nursing at a reduced entrance fee.

LEGAL POINTS

Although it may not be obvious to the nurse in training, some of the details of ward routine are based on her legal obligations to her patients; many of these points have already been mentioned, but it may be useful to summarise them here.

Patient's property.—It is usual for hospital authorities to issue instructions to all grades of staff to the effect that they cannot be responsible for the patient's personal belongings during his stay in hospital, unless these are specifically handed over for safe keeping. This fact must be brought to the patient's notice when he is admitted; should he wish to hand over money or other property (clothes), a list must be made which the patient must sign; if neither he nor his relatives are able to sign, then two nurses should check the list together and both sign. Care must be taken when describing such objects as jewellery, since it is difficult for the nurse to tell imitation stones or metal from the real thing.

When the patient is discharged, his property is returned to him and he is asked to sign a receipt.

On the death of a patient, small belongings are usually given to the relatives; should large sums of money or valuable articles be involved, the nurse should refer the matter to the administrative officer.

Consent forms.—Most hospital consent forms are so worded as to cover any procedure found to be necessary at the time of operation and also to the administration of an anaesthetic. Should any difficulties arise the surgeon must be informed. It is only in extreme emergencies that he will operate without written consent.

Prior to gynaecological operations, it is customary for the surgeon to interview the husband with a view to obtaining his consent as well as that of his wife.

For patients under the age of consent, the consent of the parent or guardian is obtained. In the case of a young person between the ages of 16 and the age of consent, should the next of kin not be available, his own signature will be recognised.

Injury to patients.—All members of the hospital staff have a responsibility to make the patients' environment as safe as possible—for example, seeing that stairs and dark passages are well lighted and that all furniture and equipment is well maintained.

Any accidents which do occur must be reported in detail while the incident is fresh in the observer's mind; the doctor must be informed and any complaints of pain or discomfort brought to his notice. In fact, this last applies to all such complaints made by patients under all circumstances, and it is a wise practice to have a written record for future reference.

It is often thought that the ward sister is legally responsible for all the happenings on her ward and this is true inasmuch as she delegates responsibility to members of her staff; this does not mean, however, that a nurse in training could not also be held responsible for negligence in some matter for which she had received adequate instruction and previous supervision.

Gifts from patients.—It is wise not to accept gifts from patients; but in the case of small personal items refusal may be difficult and may in fact upset a grateful patient. Some hospitals have strict rules on this matter and the nurse should be aware of those which exist at her training school. If money is offered, the nurse can tactfully suggest that it is given to the hospital for nurses' or patients' amenity funds, but should never accept it for herself.

Information.—Each hospital has regulations as to how information relating to patients is supplied. All queries about the patient's treatment or progress should be referred to the nurse in charge; if statements are required for the press, these are usually issued by the administrative officer of the hospital.

The nurse must also remember that it is unwise and unethical to discuss her patients outside the hospital. When she has received a confidence from a patient, she should treat it as such unless it has a direct bearing on his condition, when she should report it to the ward sister.

Patients' Wills.—Occasionally a patient is anxious to make his will; if this happens, the fact must be reported to the administrative staff, who will make suitable arrangements. In the event of a nurse being asked to witness a will, she should at once contact the Central Nursing Office for guidance. It is, however, important that the patient is able to complete his will without undue delay.

Nursing ethics involve many important principles which go beyond the letter of the law and are international rather than local. They are best summarised by quoting the International Code of Nursing Ethics as adopted by the Grand Council of the International Council of Nurses in 1953 and as revised in 1965.

INTERNATIONAL COUNCIL OF NURSES CODE OF NURSING ETHICS

1. The fundamental responsibility of the nurse is threefold: to conserve life, to alleviate suffering and to promote health.
2. The nurse must maintain at all times the highest standards of nursing care and of professional conduct.
3. The nurse must not only be well prepared to practise, but must maintain her knowledge and skill at a consistently high level.
4. The religious beliefs of a patient must be respected.

5. Nurses hold in confidence all personal information entrusted to them.
6. Nurses recognise not only the responsibilities but the limitations of their professional functions; do not recommend or give medical treatment without medical orders except in emergencies, and report such action to a physician as soon as possible.
7. The nurse is under an obligation to carry out the physician's orders intelligently and loyally and to refuse to participate in unethical procedures.
8. The nurse sustains confidence in the physician and other members of the health team; incompetence or unethical conduct of associates should be exposed, but only to the proper authority.
9. A nurse is entitled to just remuneration and accepts only such compensation as the contract, actual or implied, provides.
10. Nurses do not permit their names to be used in connection with the advertisement of products, or with any other forms of self-advertisement.
11. The nurse co-operates with and maintains harmonious relationships with members of other professions and with nursing colleagues.
12. The nurse adheres to standards of personal ethics which reflect credit upon the profession.
13. In personal conduct nurses should not knowingly disregard the accepted patterns of behaviour of the community in which they live and work.
14. The nurse participates and shares responsibility with other citizens and other health professions in promoting efforts to meet the health needs of the public—local, state, national and international.

Reference

SPELLER, S. R. (1969). *Law Notes for Nurses*. (London, Royal College of Nursing.)

INDEX

215

X

X-rays, 98
   of biliary apparatus, 99
    bronchial tree, 100
    chest, 98
    circulatory system, 99
    digestive tract, 98
    urinary tract, 99
    ventricles of brain, 100

Y

Yellowness of skin, 89
Young's rule, 193

Z

Zinc, 64